Dermatology and Allergology

Principles and Practice

Dermatology and Allergology – Principles and Practice

Publisher: iConcept Press Ltd.
Cover design: Pineapple Design Ltd.
Interior design: iConcept Press Ltd.
Typesetting and copy editing: iConcept Press Ltd. and Pineapple Design Ltd.

ISBN: 978-1-922227-95-9

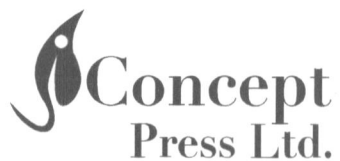

iConcept
Press Ltd.

www.iconceptpress.com

Contents

Preface

Dermatology is the branch of medicine dealing with the skin and its diseases, a unique specialty with both medical and surgical aspects. Allergology is the study of allergy and hypersensitivity, in which allergy is a hypersensitivity disorder of the immune system and hypersensitivity (also called hypersensitivity reaction or intolerance) refers to undesirable reactions produced by the normal immune system. Dermatology and allergology are two highly interrelated disciplines. *Dermatology and Allergology – Principles and Practice* provides some latest research and concerns in these two areas.

There are totally 8 chapters in this book. Chapter 1 discusses dermatologic disease with psychiatric manifestations, dermatologic disease influenced by psychosocial stress and psychiatric disorders with cutanous manifestations. Medical Illness with neuropsychiatric and dermatological manifestations and psychiatric side effects of dermatological treatment is also discussed. Chapter 2 describes the ocular surface defence and allergological mechanism when the ocular surface is introduced to foreign bodies, and reviews foreign body reaction caused by synthetic and organic fibers. Chapter 3 discusses podoconiosis, which is a debilitating disease common in several countries across the world. Unfortunately, despite its huge socioeconomic and public health burden, podoconiosis has remained neglected in clinical, public health, and policy agendas until quite recently. Chapter 4 evaluates with a second generation antihistamine, like rupatadine, the overall efficacy in the control of morning (AM) and evening (PM) nasal symptoms in patients with allergic rhinitis. This analysis includes the pooled data from five randomized, double blind, placebo-controlled studies. The findings were that overall efficacy (T4SS) relief of symptoms was quite similar for AM or PM period with rupatadine 10 mg once daily, indicating a sustained 24-hour effect of rupatadine irrespective of time of dosing.

Chapter 5 proposes to evaluate occupational and environmental risk factors for allergic and hypersensitivity reactions with a public health view. Based on the epidemiological data in developed and developing countries, the authors aim to draw attention to the current status and new ways of understanding allergies and propose solutions for the future. Chapter 6 recites the importance of clinical history for the diagnosis of anaphylaxis, validity of recent investigations/tests in lieu of anaphylaxis and interpretation of various test in the background of clinical history of anaphylaxis. Chapter 7 discusses a common nonscarring, autoimmune disease that can affect any hair-bearing area called Alopecia areata (AA). AA occurs in all ethnic groups, ages, and both sexes and may affect a small area of scalp (patchy type), or involve the entire scalp (alopecia totalis) or whole body (alopecia universalis). Chapter 8 proposes ways of targeting the mycobacterial toxin mycolactone in treatment of Buruli ulcers. Mycolactone plays a central role in ulcer formation by acting on the host at cellular and subcellular levels via several mechanisms.

Editing and publishing a book is never an easy task. Each chapter in this book has gone through a peer review, a selection and an editing process so as to guarantee its quality. Without the supports and contributions of the authors and reviewers, this book can never be able to complete. We would like to thank all of the authors in this book and all of the reviewers who participated in the reviewing process: Palok Aich, Mohammed M. H. Al-Gayyar, Ayad K Ali, Mostafa Amr, Yaakub Azhany, Nooshin Bagherani, Ola Bakry, Philippe Bégin, Denise Carmona Cara, Salvatore Chirumbolo, Mohamed El-Khalawany, Aylin Türel Ermertcan, Eckart Haneke, Martin Himly, Mark R. Hutchinson, Victor J. Johnson, Choun-Ki Joo, Osmo Kari, Ujendra Kumar, Hoàng Thị Lâm, Jere J. Mammino, Peizhong Mao, Ian A. Myles, Kazue Nakanaga, Ellen Namork, Yoichiro Okubo, Arnold P. Oranje, Kyoung-Chan Park, Girolamo Pelaia, T. S. Sathyanarayana Rao, Lidia Rudnicka, Amin Saburi, Silvia Solís-Ortiz, Paolo Sossai, Ozlem Su, Sherif S. Sultan, HaiLun Sun, Hajime Takizawa, Gaurav Tomar and Viroj Wiwanitkit. We hope that you, the reader, will find this book interesting and useful. Any advices please feel free and are always welcome to tell us.

iConcept Press Ltd
September 2014

Psychodermatology: An Update

Suprakash Chaudhury

Department of Psychiatry
Rural Medical College and Pravara Rural Hospital
Pravara Institute of Medical Sciences (Deemed University), Loni, India

1   Introduction

Psychodermatology or Psychocutaneous medicine straddles the interface of psychiatry and dermatology. Estimates of dermatological and psychiatric co-morbidity are high, ranging from 30% to 60% (Korabel *et al.*, 2008; Orion & Ben-Avi, 2011). Understanding the psychosocial and occupational context of skin disease is critical for the optimal management of psychocutaneous disorders. Correlation between psychiatric and dermatological disorders exists due to more than a fact, that the brain, as the center of psychological functions, and the skin has the same ectodermal origin. Connecting the two disciplines is a complex interplay between neuroendocrine and immune systems that has been described as the NICS, or the neuro-immuno-cutaneous system. The interaction between nervous system, skin and immunity has been explained by release of mediators from NICS (Yadav *et al.*, 2013) (Figure1). It is a highly complex relation considering etiology, diagnostic procedures and treatment. Liaison therapy enables multidisciplinary approach with the cooperation of psychiatric and dermatologic teams and simultaneous diagnostic procedures and the treatment of patients with psychocutaneous disorders. Survey among psychiatrists and dermatologists has shown that knowledge about the diagnosis, treatment and/or appropriate referral for psychocutaneous disorders is lacking (Jafferany *et al.*, 2010a; Jafferany *et al.*, 2010b). Significant information gaps were also identified in the knowledge of patient or family resources on psydermatological disorders. This can be only be rectified by incorporating formal training and didactics on psychodermatology in dermatology and psychiatry residency programs and regular CME events (Jafferany*et al.*, 2010a; Jafferany*et al.*, 2010b).

2   Classification of Psychocutaneous Phenomena

2.1 Dermatological Disease with Psychiatric Manifestations (Secondary Psychiatric Disorders)

This category includes patients who have emotional problems as a result of having skin disease. Symptoms of depression and anxiety, work-related problems and impaired social interactions are frequently observed. Fundamentally, dermatological diseases are in this group, but these diseases are strongly influenced by psychosomatic factors. Although the etiology of the disease is physiological, psychological factors and stress exacerbate the dermatological symptoms and psychosocial effects of the diseases increase stress. The most important variable that results in psychological susceptibility in dermatological diseases is deformation. The magnitude of this effect is closely related to patients' relationships between self-perception and others (Alopecia areata, Chronic eczema, Cystic acne, Hemangiomas, Ichthyosis, Psoriasis, Vitiligo, Rhinophyma, Melasma, Androgenetic alopecia, Hirsuitism, Scars/keloids, Kaposi's sarcoma).

2.2   Dermatological diseases influenced by psychosocial stress (Psychophysiological disorders)

The etiology of the disease is, again, multifactorial. On the one hand, stressful situations, and on the other hand, complex physiological and psychological defense mechanisms attract attention. The relationship between dermatosis and psychological conditions is least understood in this group. While looking for the organic causes, psychological reasons should also be considered in these patients. There are various theories about the complicated mechanisms that cause diseases. Psychoneuroimmunological factors have a

Various Stress producing stimuli

Psychological: Anxiety, depression, anger, frustration and helplessness
Environmental: Heat or cold, noise, pollutants, UV light, mechanical damage, high/low humidity, allergens
Behavioural: Isolation, overcrowding, physical restraint, enforced starvation, change in diet, job strain, burnout, unemployment and refugee status

HPA axis & Autonomic nervous system activation

↑CRH, ACTH, PRL

Sympathetic nervous system activation

↑ Substance P
CGRP, VIP
Neuropeptide Y
Somatostatins
Neurokins A and B
Opiomelanocortins

Lymphocytosis & their activation

CRH, Growth Factors (NGF,SCF) released

Skin mast cell activation

CRH-R receptor on Mast cell activated

Supresses TH1 immune response
Upregulates TH2 immune response
↑ Skin serotonin level

Immune dysregulation
Neurogenic inflammation
Proinflammatory response
Vasodilation

Inflammatory
Autoimmune
Allergic skin disorders

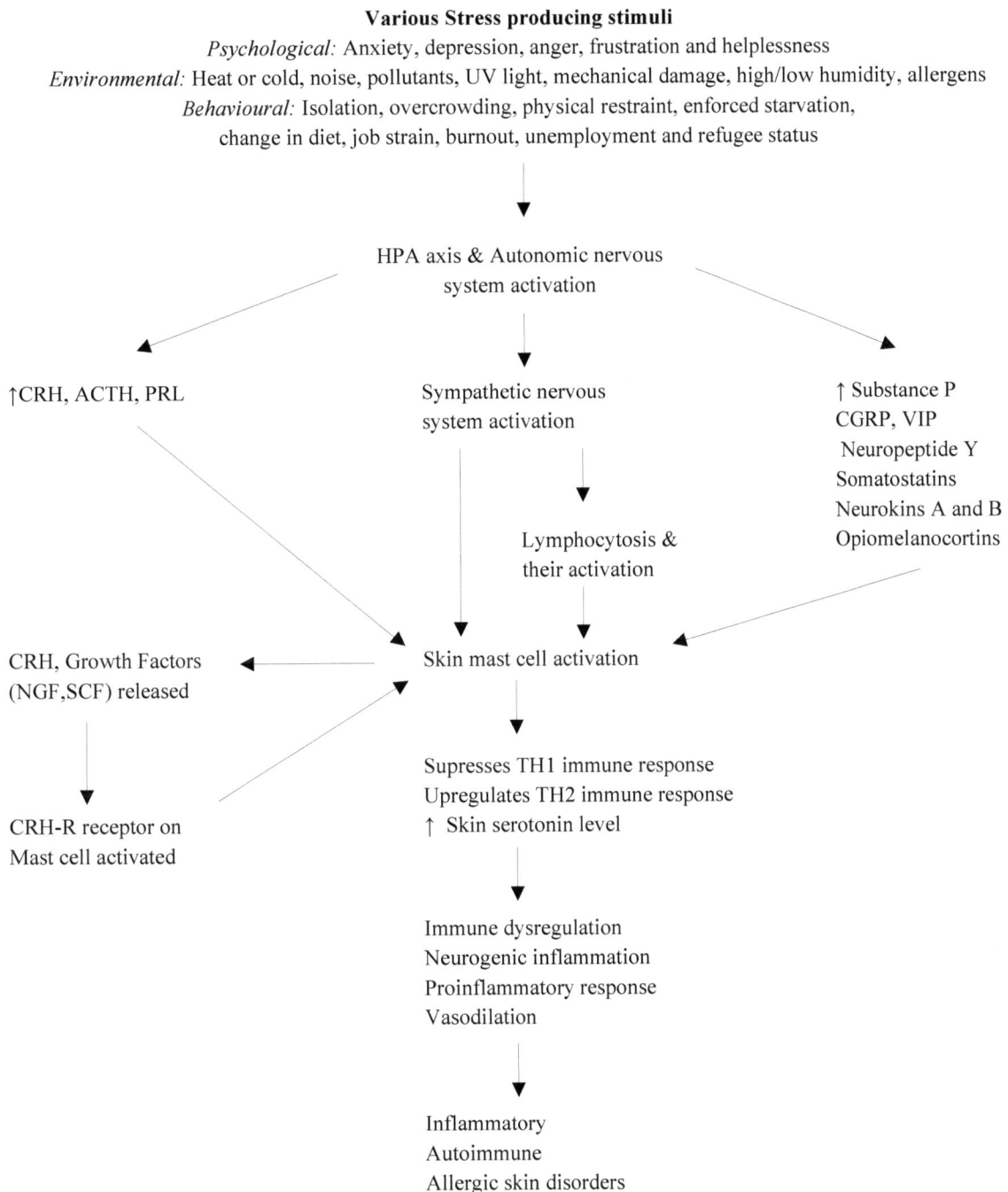

Figure1: Interplay of various factors leading to psychocutaneous disorders (Modified from Yadav et al,2013). ACTH: Adrenocorticotrophic hormone; CGRP: calcitonin gene related peptide; CRH: corticotrophin releasing hormone, CRH-R: CRH receptor; HPA: Hypothalamus pituitary adrenal ; NGF: Nerve growth factor; PRL: Prolactin; SCF: stem cell factor; Th: T helper; VIP: vasoactive intestinal peptide.

role in the majority of diseases. Patients in this group are the most difficult to treat (Acne, Alopecia areata, Atopic dermatitis, Psoriasis, Psychogenic purpura, Rosacea, Seborrheic dermatitis, Urticaria (hives)).

2.3 Psychiatric Disorders with Cutaneous Manifestations (Primary Psychiatric Disorders)

In this group, the underlying cause of symptoms is psychiatric but when these patients present to a dermatologist, they deny their psychopathologies and want to be treated by the dermatologist. Directly destroying the defenses of these patients and referring them to psychiatry is harmful because of the possibility of suicidal intentions or the appearance of severe psychiatric conditions. Brief and frequent dermatology consultations let the patient develop a good relationship, making the passage to psychiatry easier (Delusions of parasitosis, Bromosiderophobia, Dysmorphophobia, Factitial dermatitis, Neurotic excoriations, Trichotillomania, Somatoform pain disorders, Psychogenic purpura, Eating disorders).

SLE: malar erythematous rash, discoid rash, patchy alopecia, photosensitivity, other rashes (maculopapular, urticarial, bullous), vasculitis (nodules, ulcers, purpura, infarcts).

Essential mixed cryoglobulinemia: urticaria, palpable purpura, ecchymoses, macules & papules, nodules, vesicles and bullae, necrotic ulcerations

Hyperthyroidism: increased sweating, warm moist skin, fine hair, hair loss.

Hypothyroidism: cool dry skin, edema, hair loss

Cushing's syndrome: purple striae, excessive bruising, acne, hirsuitism, edema

Addison's disease: hyperpigmentation

Porphyria: blisters, abrasions, hyperpigmentations, hypertrichosis, photosensitivity

AIDS: Kaposis sarcoma, seborrheic dermatitis, pruritus, other manifestations of opportunistic infections (e.g. herpes, candidiasis, syphilis).

Table 1: Medical Illness with Neuropsychiatric and Dermatological manifestations

---

Steroids: depression, hypomania, mania, delirium, acute delusions, hallucinations.

Isotretinoin: depression, suicidal thoughts and even suicidal attempts.

Rifampicin: drowsiness, dizziness, confusion, behavioral changes, cognitive disturbances, delusions, hallucinations.

Dapsone: insomnia

Acyclovir: aggression, delirium, hallucinations, depression, psychosis.

Chloroquin: fatigue, personality changes.

Cetrizine: drwsiness, dizziness, insomnia, nervousness, irritability, depersonalization, depression.

Fexofenadine: insomnia, nervousness, sleep disorders, terrifying dreams.

Zidovudine: insomnia, agitation.

Table 2: Psychiatric side effects of Dermatological treatment

Lithium: macupapular and urticarial eruptions; alopecia (diffuse or localized); increase in verrucous growths (warts); precipitation and exacerbation of psoriasis and acne; folliculitis; lupus like syndrome; exacerbation of Darier's disease (keratosis follicularis); nail pigmentation; exfoliative dermatitis.

Antipsychotics: skin pigmentation changes (especiallyphenothiazines, thioridazine, haloperidol, clozapine, perphenazine); photosensitivity; lupus like syndrome (especially chlorpromazine, thioridazine, perphenazine); hypersensitivity reactions (urticaria, macupapular eruptions, petechiae, and edema); contact dermatitis (especially with oral suspension or solution of thioridazine, haloperidol or fluphenazine); injection site reaction with haloperidol decanoate; seborrheic dermatitis; erythema multiforme, Stevens-Johnson syndrome, nonthrombocytopenic purpura; urticaria; palmar erythema.

Antidepressants: allergic reactions including urticaria, macular or maculopapular skin rash; petechiae; leukonychia, angioedema, purpura and exfoliative dermatitis; erythema multiforme (reported with trazodoneplus lithium, sertraline and fluoxetine); serum sickness (with fluoxetine); photosensitivity (with tricyclic antidepressants); leukocytoplastic vasculitis (with trazodone, maprotiline or fluoxetine); acne (with maprotiline; pustular psoriasis with trazodone); alopecia (with imipramine and fluoxetine); pathologic sweating.

Anticonvulsants: *Carbamazepine* pruritic rashes, exfoliative dermatitis, systemic lupus erythematosus, hair loss, erythema multiforme and Steven-Johnson syndrome, hypersensitivity reactions characterized by a generalized skin rash, lymphadenopathy and fever.

Valproic acid associated with hair loss, changing hair colour, scleroderma, cutaneous vaculitis and systemic lupus erythematosis.

Lamotrigine maculopapular &/or erythematous eruptions, Steven-Johnson syndrome, toxic epidermal necrolysis, angioedema, and a rash associated with a variable number of systemic features including fever, lymphadenopathy, facial swelling, hematologic and hepatologic abnormalities.

Gabapentine associated with alopecia.

Anxiolytics: Benzodiazepines associated with mild generalized skin rash. Photosensitivity reported with chlordiazepoxide and alprazolam. Hyperpigmentation at sites of dermabrasion with diazepam. Bullous lesions after overdose of diazepam. Exacerbation of porphyria; urticaria; erythema multiforme, erythema nodosum.

Methylphenidate: eryhtema multiforme, exfoliative dermatitis, hair loss, rash, urticaria.

Atomoxatine: dermatitis.

Rivastigmine: urticaria, Stevens-Johnson syndrome

Modafinil: dry skin

Naltrexone: skin rash

Table 3: Cutaneous side effects of psychotropic medications

3   Dermatological Disease with Psychiatric Manifestations

The psychosocial effect of skin diseases is considerable and unappreciated. Although skin conditions are usually not life-threatening, because of their visibility they can be "life-ruining." Persons with disfigurement frequently feel psychologically and socially devastated as a result. Moreover, persons with skin disorders have trouble getting jobs in which appearance is important (Ginsburg & Link, 1993).It is also well documented that persons with visible disfigurement face discrimination, especially if the condition is perceived to be contagious (Love *et al.*, 1987). There are certain findings which explain high co-morbidity of cutaneous and psychiatric disorders:

   a) Chronic skin disease involves life adaptation which, in most cases, results in lower life quality, influencing patient's social life and making the treatment more difficult

b) Noticeability of skin lesions exposes the patient to negative society reactions and stigmatization because of disfigurement, resulting in patient's loss of self-confidence

c) Factors like severe anxiety, emotional instability and loss of self –confidence reduce the quality of life and working abilities in such patients.

Assessment of the impact of skin disease on patients' lives revealed that 29% of cases had symptoms of depression and 61% had symptoms of anxiety and felt that they had a lack of spontaneity. Forty percent of cases felt that their social lives were impaired due to the skin disease and 64% indicated that they had work-related problems due to the skin disease (Jowett & Ryan, 1985). The most common findings on assessment of patients with dermatologic disease using psychiatric rating scales are high scores on depression and anxiety (Chaudhury & Das, 1998a, 1998b; Chaudhury et al., 1993). The skin diseases most frequently implicated with co-morbid psychiatric diagnoses are eczema, psoriasis and acne vulgaris (Barankin & Dekoven, 2002).Alexithymia is a personality trait characterized by difficulties in differentiating and describing feelings. Preliminary data show that alexithymia is associated with alopecia areata, psoriasis, atopic dermatitis, vitiligo and chronic urticaria. Besides treating comorbid psychological problems such as anxiety and depression, dermatologists should also be aware of alexithymia and its possible association with an underlying dermatologic disease (Chaudhury & Das, 1998a; Willemsen et al, 2008).

3.1 Acne

Skin conditions, such as acne, are sometimes thought of as insignificant in comparison with diseases of other organ systems. Physicians' assumptions about the effects of a skin condition are often inaccurate. The psychological effect of acne is unique for each patient. Patients should be asked how much their acne bothers them, regardless of how severe it appears to physicians. Acne's effect on psychosocial and emotional problems, however, is comparable to that of arthritis, back pain, diabetes, epilepsy, and disabling asthma (Mallon et al., 1999).Acne vulgaris often flares with stress and premenstrually. With worsening of the acne, many individuals get more stressed, setting up a vicious cycle (Shenefelt, 2010). Acne has a demonstrable association with depression and anxiety; it affects personality, emotions, self-image and esteem, less satisfaction with general appearance, feelings of social isolation, social impairment and lower quality of life (Barankin & Dekoven, 2002;Mallonet al., 1999). Its substantial influence is likely related to its typical appearance on the face, and would help explain the increased unemployment rate of adults with acne. Because the face is so important to body image, young men with severe scarring acne are at particular risk of depression and suicide (Cotterill & Cunliffe, 1997).A population based study of 3775 adolescents, including 493 suffering from self-declared substantial acne observed that suicidal ideation was reported by only 9.5% of those with no acne or little acne, 18.6%of those with moderate acne, and 24.1%of those with substantial acne (odds ratio approximately 2). The differences were greater in boys than in girls (Halvorsen et al, 2011).Acne appears to be an independent risk factor for suicidal ideation, especially in boys (Misery, 2011).Poor self-concept, perfectionist and compulsive personality traits, correlated more strongly with self-excoriative behavior than the dermatologic indices of acne severity, suggesting that psychological factors, independent of acne severity, play an important role in the perpetuation of the self-excoriative behavior exhibited by some women with acne (Gupta et al, 1996).

Much of the disability caused by acne can be reduced with appropriate medical treatment. Interventions, such as isotretinoin, that minimize or prevent scarring and reduce duration of the condition have the most pronounced psychosocial benefit (Misery *et al.*, 2012).Stress reduction techniques like relaxation training, biofeedback, meditation, or self-hypnosis may be helpful (Shenefelt, 2010).

3.2   Atopic dermatitis (AD)

AD is a complex disease traditionally involving interaction of genetic, environmental, and immunologic factors. Recent studies suggest psycho-neuro-immunologic factors and emotional stress are important in its evolution. The observations that internal (bacterial infections) or external(psychologic) stressors may induce AD flares is explained by studies showing that stress impairs the skin barrier function and favors a shift in immunity toward a T helper type 2 cell/allergic response. Furthermore, those with AD appear to have an inherited hypothalamic deficiency that impairs normal hypothalamic-pituitary-adrenal axis function. Neuropeptides released in the skin may also mediate neurogenic inflammation, including mast cell degranulation. AD causes significant stress and impaired quality of life in patients and their family members (Arndt *et al*, 2008).

When AD affects infants, skin sensation is often altered, which can result in impaired emotional development because the skin is critical in sensory perception and communication. Skin contact between infants and parents contributes not only to infants' learning their boundaries, but also positively affects the attitudes of caregivers; this serves to generate feelings of well-being and self-esteem (Koblenzer, 1996). AD can cause many sleepless nights for children, and therefore also their parents. It can also interfere with school performance and social relationships. One study found twice the rate of psychological disturbance among children with moderately severe and severe AD as among a control group (Absolon*et al*, 1997). Parents of infants and children with this condition often are anxious, frustrated, and angry both with their children and with their physicians. Providing a few extra minutes to empathize with a patient's or parents' unique situation can help a strained therapeutic relationship.

The onset or exacerbation of atopic dermatitis often follows stressful life events (Picardi & Abeni, 2001). Adult patients with this condition can have substantial salary loss from missed work, as well as large expenditures for emollients, topical steroids, clothing and bedding, laundry, and possibly consultation with alternative medicine practitioners. Along with the financial strain, patients are often concerned about personal appearance, attractiveness, career aspirations, and the ability to form personal relationships. Impaired sexual function through both physical and psychological mechanisms can compound the adverse effects (Barankin & Dekoven, 2002; Gil, 2006).Adults with AD are often anxious and depressed with problems in psychosocial adjustment and low self-esteem (Lapidus & Kerr, 2001;Bockelbrink*et al*, 2006; Hashizume *et al*, 2005;Gupta & Gupta, 2003).Psychological and stress-reduction interventions significantly improve cutaneous manifestations and patient well-being (Arndt *etal*, 2008). Stress may be lessened with cognitive behavioral therapy, hypnosis or self hypnosis. Anxiolytics and antidepressants are employed for treatment of anxiety and depression respectively (Shenefelt, 2010).

3.3   Psoriasis

Psoriasis has a substantial effect on patients' lives and can greatly increase the risk of suicide. Patients are often most troubled by the itching and scratching, bleeding, unsightly physical appearance, and noticeable flakes. The degree of pruritus in patients with psoriasis and AD is strongly correlated to depressive psychopathology. Both physical and mental functioning are reduced in patients with psoriasis comparable to that in arthritis, cancer, depression, and heart disease patients (Rapp *et al*, 1999). In a study of 369 patients with psoriasis, 35% reported that their condition affected their careers; 20% reported that they were substantially impaired in performing their work (Finlay & Coles, 1995).Quality of life may be severely affected by the chronicity and visibility of psoriasis as well as by the need for lifelong treatment. Five dimensions of the stigma associated with psoriasis have been identified: (1) Anticipation of rejection, (2) feelings of being flawed, (3) sensitivity to the attitudes of society, (4) guilt and shame and (5) secretiveness (Ginsburg & Link, 1999).

Depressive symptoms and suicidal ideation is frequently associated in psoriasis (Schmitt & Ford, 2007; Esposito, 2006).Many have feelings of physical and sexual unattractiveness as well as helplessness, anger, and frustration. Shame or embarrassment with resultant secretiveness and avoidance of common social activities, like sports and swimming is not unusual. The disease is clearly associated with increased alcohol consumption and smoking (Herron *et al*, 2005).

Even though the emotional effects and functional impact of the disease are not necessarily proportionate to the clinical severity of psoriasis (Russo *et al*, 2004), the frequency of psychiatric disturbance decreases with improvement in the clinical severity and symptoms of psoriasis (Sampogna *et al*, 2007).The effect of the disease decreases with increasing age, probably a function of both disease duration and a more settled lifestyle. Women appear to report greater impairment of quality of life, while men report greater work-related stresses. While the severity of the condition can influence psychosocial well-being, it is important to appreciate that people perceive their conditions differently, such that those with only mild psoriasis can in fact be more bothered than those with extensive, severe disease. A questionnaire based study on 300 patients with moderate to severe chronic plaque psoriasis from 17 dermatology clinics throughout Italy revealed that psoriasis elicited anger, annoyance, and irritation in approximately 50% of the patients, whilst 38% of patients were unable to describe their emotional state. Aspects of life that were limited by psoriasis included clothing (57%), social interactions (43%), and personal hygiene (31%). The disease was often seen by patients as incomprehensible, incurable, and uncontrollable. More than half of the patients stressed their need to be listened to by the treating physician, and their wish that the physician should use simple language and should improve their psychological skills and interpersonal communication techniques. Dermatologists need to convey to patients with psoriasis the feeling of 'understanding the disease,' of hope about its curability, and the 'perception of control.' These elements should be taken into account when treating patients and whenever educational interventions are planned (Linder *et al*, 2009).

Proper medical treatment of psoriasis is important because it improves patients' lives. The treatment itself can also affect quality of life based on efficacy, convenience, discomfort, and time commitment. In 40% to 80% of patients with psoriasis, stress is reported to influence onset and progression of the condition; direct and indirect suppression of the immune system is the most likely etiology (Barankin & Dekoven, 2002). Body image issues and stress may be improved with cognitive behavioral therapy, biofeedback, meditation, relaxation training or self-hypnosis. Self-hypnosis can reduce pruritusor itching and give a sense of greater self-control, which in turn can lessen the depression (Shenefelt, 2010).Psychological interventions and antidepressant medications may improve perceived symptom severity, quality of life and major compliance to the treatment in selected patients (suffering from psoriasis and mood disturbance), without a clinician necessarily being able to see an impact on psoriasis severity (D'Erme *et al*, 2012).

3.4 Alopecia areata (AA)

Psychologic factors may affect the development, evolution and therapeutic management of AA. Acute emotional stress may precipitate AA by activation of overexpressed type 2b corticotropin-releasing hormone receptors around the hair follicles leading to intense local inflammation (Katsarou-Katsari *et al*, 2001).Release of substance P from peripheral nerves in response to stress, and prominent substance P expression in nerves surrounding hair follicles has been reported in AA patients (Toyoda *et al*, 2001). Substance P degrading enzyme neutral endopeptidase has also been strongly expressed in affected hair follicles in the acute-progressive as well as the chronic-stable phase of the disorder (Toyoda *et al*, 2001). The hair loss can aggravate the stress, especially if the hair loss is visible to others (Shenefelt, 2010).Alexithymia and dissociative somatization was more common in adults with AA than in controls (Williamson *et al*, 2009). Comorbid psychiatric disorders are common and include major depression, generalized anxiety disorder, phobic states and paranoid disorder (Garcia-Hernandez *et al*, 1999).Self-image issues and stress may be treated with self-hypnosis (Shenefelt, 2010) or other stress reduction techniques.

3.5 Vitiligo

Stress can exacerbate vitiligo by changing immune function, increasing production of opioid peptides, increasing catecholamine release, and affecting other hormone pathways. Vitiligoin turn causes disfigurement, leading to increase in anxiety, embarrassment, self-consciousness and psychiatric morbidity along with low self-esteem (Lee& Koo, 2003). Younger patients and individuals in lower socioeconomic groups show poor adjustment, low self-esteem and problems with social adaptation (Porter *et al*, 1979; Koshevenko, 1989). Most patients with vitiligo report a negative impact on sexual relationships and cite embarrassment as the cause (Porter *et al*, 1990).

Psychiatric morbidity is typically reported in approximately one-third of patients (Padopoulos *et al*, 1998), but, in one study, 56% of the sample had adjustment disorder and 29% had depressive disorders (Mattoo *et al*, 2001).In depression-prone individuals, vitiligo can initiate or exacerbate depression, especially in darkly pigmented individuals (Dogra & Kanawar, 2002). The prevalence of depression in vitiligo patients was 39% in a recent quality of life study (Sampogna *et al*, 2008). Depression may be treated by antidepressants and cognitive-behavioral therapy (Papadopoulos *et al*, 1999).Hypnosis can also help to reframe the patient's perspective on their depigmented lesions, lessening secondary depression (Shenefelt, 2010).

4 Dermatological Disease Influenced by Psychosocial Stress

Psychophysiologic disorders rcfcr to those cases of bona fide skin disorder, such as urticaria, psoriasis, acne, AA, AD and rosacea that can be exacerbated by emotional stress in the patient. It is important to note that these disorders are not "caused" by stress, but are simply exacerbated by stress (Table 4) (Griesemer, 1978). Each of these conditions has "stress responders" and "non-stress responders," depending on whether a patient's skin disease is or is not frequently and predictably exacerbated by stress. In examining distressed patients with flare-up of a real skin disorder such as eczema, it is important to determine how much of the emotional distress is psychosomatic and how much of it is somatopsychic in nature. A psychosomatic problem refers to a situation whereby external stresses such as occupational difficulty or family problems lead to worsening of the skin disease. Sometimes, both psychosomatic and somatopsychic elements may be active in creating a vicious cycle that perpetuates the flare up of the skin disease. It has been estimated that the effective management of at least one-third of patients attending skin departments depends to some extent upon the recognition of emotional factors.

4.1   Chronic urticaria

Like anychronic disease, it raises two principal problems: preservation of the quality of life and therapeutic compliance. In chronic urticaria, psychological factors intervene on several levels: the doctor-patient relationship, the urticarian crisis itself, the onset and/or the aggravation of the disease, and thepsychosocial consequences of urticaria. The role of psychological factors in the onset and/or the aggravation of the disease are variously estimated, without consensus between the authors. Severe emotional stress may exacerbate preexisting urticaria (Rees, 1957). Increased emotional tension, fatigue, and stressful life situations may be primary factors in more than 20% of cases and are contributory in 68% of patients. Difficulties with expression of anger and a need for approvals from others are also common (Juhlin, 1981). Patients with this disorder may have symptoms of depression and anxiety, and the severity of pruritus appears to increase as the severity of depression increases (Gupta *et al*, 1994; Shiro *et al*, 1994).Quality of life is especially impaired. Treatments of chronic urticaria should combine dermatological treatment with prescription of psychotropic drugs (especially antidepressants), along with psychotherapy (a relaxation technique for example), without forgetting health education sessions (Consoli, 2003). Self-hypnosis can reduce pruritus or itching and give a sense of greater self-control, which can lessen the depression. Hypnosis has resolved some cases of chronic urticaria (Shenefelt, 2010).

Diagnosis	Proportion with emotional trigger (%)
Hyperhydrosis	100
Lichen simplex chronicus	98
Rosacea	94
Dyshidrosis	76
Atopic dermatitis	70
Urticaria	68
Psoriasis	62
Papular acne vulgaris	55
Seborrheic dermatitis	41
Fungus infection	9
Nevi	0
Basal cell carcinoma	0
Keratoses	0

Table 4: Incidence of emotional triggering of common dermatoses (N=4576) (Griesemer, 1978)

4.2   Herpes simplex

Stress frequently initiates or exacerbates herpes simplex cold sore virus recurrences (Buske-Kirchenbaum *et al*, 2001). Along with conventional antiviral treatments for the herpes, stress reduction techniques may be useful (Shenefelt, 2010).

4.3   Hyperhidrosis

Hyperhidrosis of hands, feet, axillae, or forehead is related to stress. Locally injected botulinum toxin can temporarily inactivate acetylcholine release from the nerves associated with sweating (Lowe *et al*, 2007). Stress reduction techniques including biofeedback are useful (Shenefelt, 2010).

4.4   Lichen planus

Lichen planus, an inflammatory pruritic dermatosis, is often triggered or exacerbated by stress. The intense itching and discoloration with hyperpigmentation that occur with lichen planus can further aggravate the stress. The stress may be reduced using relaxation, biofeedback, meditation, or self-hypnosis (Shenefelt, 2010).

4.5   Lichen simplex chronicus

Thickened plaques of lichen simplex chronicus are produced by rubbing or scratching the skin and are initiated or exacerbated by stress. Along with standard dermatoical treatments, stress reduction is beneficial (Shenefelt, 2010).

4.6   Seborrheic dermatitis:

The scaling and itching of seborrheic dermatitis is frequently worsened by stress (Arck&Paus, 2006). In addition to conventional treatments, stress reduction techniques like relaxation, biofeedback, meditation, or self-hypnosis may be useful (Shenefelt, 2010).

4.7   Postherpetic neuralgia

Postherpetic neuralgia is a peripheral neuropathic pruritus, pain, or paraesthesia following herpes zoster. Topical treatment with capsaicin four or five times a day, which depletes substance P in the nerves, may be useful. Oral gabapentin also may help reduce the neuropathic sensations. Acupuncture and hypnosis have provided relief from pain or pruritus in some patients (Shenefelt, 2010).

5   Psychiatric Disorders with Cutaneous Manifestations

5.1   Psychotic Disorders

5.1.1   Delusions of parasitosis

Patients with delusions of parasitosis firmly believe that their bodies are infested by some type of organism. Frequently, they have elaborate ideas about how these "organisms" mate, reproduce, move around in the skin and, sometimes, exit the skin. These patients often present with the "matchbox" sign, in which small bits of excoriated skin, debris or unrelated insects or insect parts are brought in matchboxes or other containers as "proof" of infestation (Chaudhury & Augustine, 1990). The psychiatric differential diagnosis includes schizophrenia, psychotic depression, mania with psychosis, drug-induced psychosis, and formication without delusion, in which the patient experiences crawling, biting and stinging sensations without believing that they are caused by organisms. Other organic causes such as withdrawal from cocaine, amphetamines or alcohol, vitamin B_{12} deficiency, multiple sclerosis, cerebrovascular disease or syphilis should also be considered. If any of these underlying causes are diagnosed, a separate diagnosis of delusions of parasitosis should not be made. The treatment can be very difficult. Usually the patient had already consulted a number of physicians in a variety of specialities, undergone a multitude of diagnostic studies that revealed no abnormalities and sought help from non-medical sources. The greatest challenge in the treatment of delusional patients is to obtain their trust. It is important to avoid an argument because delusional patients cannot be argued out of their delusional belief system and this will only antagonize them and sabotage the doctor - patient relationship. These patients are frequently mistrustful of physicians. They often complain that the previous physician did not examine their skin adequately. Therefore, one of the best ways to gain their trust is to give them a thorough skin examination. The treatment of choice is pimozide, a high potency antipsychotic with antipruritic properties. The medication should be presented as a "therapeutic trial," and any contentious argument regarding the pathogenesis of the disorder or the mechanism of action of pimozide should be purposely avoided. Encouragement suggesting that pimozide may "help one focus less on the skin and more on enjoying life" may help. Pimozide has been shown to be uniquely effective in the treatment of this condition, especially in decreasing formication (Srinivasan et al, 1994). Although delusional patients may agree to take psychotropic medication, they are frequently ambivalent about doing so. Therefore, if the patient should develop side effects such as stiffness or restlessness, they are liable to stop the entire treatment and never agree to take psychotropic medication again. It is important to inform patients about the side effects and to start with a low dose which is slowly titrated upward to minimize the risk of side effects. However, pimozide has a significant broad spectrum of adverse effects including extrapyramidal and cardiac side effects. Therefore, atypical antipsychotics (olanzapine, risperidone) which have considerably fewer side effects are increasingly preferred. The dosage of antipsychotic drug for treatment of delusions of parasitosis is much lower than that used for schizophrenia. Optimal therapeutic effect may not occur for 6 to 8 weeks. During the treatment course, patients become less agitated. The antipsychotic drug can be continued at the lowest effective dosage for several months and gradually tapered off without necessarily inviting the recurrence of symptoms. If the condition recurs, another course of antipsychotic therapy can be instituted.

5.1.2   Other delusional disorders, somatic type

In the delusional variant of body dysmorphic disorder, the preoccupations with a defect in appearance are of delusional intensity, although the distinction between an obsessive concern and delusion is not always clear. The disorder may respond preferentially to a selective serotonin reuptake inhibitors (SSRI), and if a patient does not completely respond to an SSRI, the addition of an antipsychotic may help. The delusion of a foul body odor (delusion of bromosis) is another encapsulated somatic delusion that a dermatologist may encounter. Treatment data are limited, but antipsychotics may be effective.

5.2   Somatoform Disorders

5.2.1   Body Dysmorphic Disorder, Dysmorphophobia or Dermatological Non-Disease

These patients are preoccupied with the idea that they are physically misshapen. This preoccupation, often involves in particular the face in women, and the scalp and genitalia in men. Facial symptoms include excessive redness, blushing, scarring, large pores, facial hair and protruding or sunken parts of face. Other symptoms are hair loss, red scrotum, urethral discharge and herpes and AIDS phobia. Strategies to relieve the anxiety due to the perceived defects may include camouflaging the lesions, mirror checking, comparison of 'defects' with the same body parts on others, questioning/reassurance seeking, mirror avoidance and grooming to cover up 'defects'(Phillips & Dufresne, 2000).Patients with body image disorders, especially those involving the face, may be suicidal (Koblenzer, 1985). Associated comorbidity in dysmorphophobia may include depression, impairment in social and occupational functioning, social phobias, OCD, skin picking, marital difficulties and substance abuse (Phillips & Dufresne, 2002).The disorder was found in 14% of dermatology outpatients and 10% of cosmetic surgery patients with a gender ratio of 1. These patients usually refuse psychiatric treatment. SSRI are effective in reducing symptoms in at least 50 percent of cases although Tricyclic Antidepressants (TCA), Mono Amino Oxidase Inhibitors (MAOI) and Pimozide have also been reported to be useful (Saini *et al*, 2004).

5.2.2   Chronic idiopathic pruritus

Although pruritus is a common and distressing symptom, its pathophysiology is not completely understood. In histamine-induced pruritus, psychic trauma lowers itch threshold, aggravates itch intensity, and prologs itch duration. Recent stressful life events have also been correlated with an increased ability to detect itch. In psoriasis, AD and chronic idiopathic urticaria a direct correlation between pruritus severity and the degree of depressive symptoms was seen, possibly due to reduced itch threshold (Gupta & Gupta, 2003). Psychiatric factors may influence the perception of itch by several mechanisms. The hypothalamus and other components of the limbic system may modulate sensory perception through the sensory cortex, and elevation of corticotrophin releasing hormone in some depressed patients may increase central nervous system opiate levels, enhancing the perception of pruritus. Neuropeptides, such as substance P, released in response to stress also produce itching. Chronic idiopathic pruritus and idiopathic pruritus ani, idiopathic pruritus vulvae, and idiopathic pruritus scroti have frequently been called psychogenic, but more study is needed to determine how psychiatric and other CNS disorders contribute to the development of pruritus. Antidepressant medications, particularly TCAs, can relieve pruritus of many origins. Behavioral treatment aimed at interrupting the itch-scratch cycle may also be important.

5.2.3   Somatoform Pain Disorder

Glossodynia

Glossodynia (burning mouth syndrome) is an unexplained prolonged sensation of pain or burning inside the oral cavity, most frequently at the tip and lateral borders of the tongue, along with dryness, paraesthesia, and changes in taste and smell. Psychiatric factors like anxiety, depression and stressful life events play a role in many patients with glossodynia. In open trials antidepressants (TCAs, SSRIs and MAOIs) and benzodiazepines have shown beneficial effects. Gabapentine may be an option.

Vulvodynia

Vulvodynia is a chronic vulvar and perineal discomfort of variable severity with burning, stinging, irritation and rawness. It is postulated that essential or dysesthetic vulvodynia results from a problem with cutaneous perception, either centrally or at the nerve root. It is more frequent in perimenopausal or postmenopausal women and is characterized by constant vulvar or perineal discomfort, as well as frequent urethral and rectal discomfort. Patients may respond to treatment with TCAs. Gabapentin may be an alternative.

5.3   Obsessive-Compulsive Spectrum Disorders

5.3.1   Psychogenic excoriations

Psychogenic excoriations (Neurotic excoriations, acne excoriee, pathological or compulsive skin picking, and dermatotillomania): is characterized by excessive scratching or picking of normal skin or skin with some inconsequential irregularity e.g. insect bite, folliculitis or acne. The distribution is bilateral, symmetrical, and accessible to the fingers; most commonly, lesions are on the face, upper back, chest, and extremities. Lesions are present in all stages of evolution and may range from small circular crusted papules to deep craters with hypertrophic borders. The skin picking is an impulsive reaction and does not belong to the obsessive-compulsive spectrum disorders: impulsivity is defined by ineffective or failing control resulting in uninhibited behavior (Misery *et al*, 2012).Co-morbid depressive and anxiety disorders are common (Calikusu et al, 2003). Patients respond to treatment with doxepin, clomipramine, and SSRIs. There are case reports of successful treatment with olanzapine, pimozide, naltrexone and behavioral therapy.

5.3.2   Trichotillomania

Trichotillomaniais a condition in which a person pulls out his or her own hair. The peak onset is in childhood with a female to male ratio of 5:1. Hair is plucked in a wave-like pattern from a single point, either in ever-expanding circles or from front to back. Though eyebrows, eyelashes, pubic or torso hair may be plucked, scalp hair is the most common. The scalp itself is normal, but within the patch the hairs are sparse and of differing lengths, depending on the phase in the plucking cycle. The extracted hair may also be chewed or swallowed (trichophagia), leading to trichobezoars (Chaudhury*et al*, 2001; Chaudhury*et al*, 2003).The most common underlying psychopathology is obsessive-compulsive disorder. The other possible underlying psychiatric diagnoses include simple habit disorder, reaction to situational stress, mental retardation, anxiety, mood disorder, substance use, eating disorder and delusions in which the patient pulls out his or her hair based on a delusional belief that something in the roots needs to be 'dug out' so the hair can grow normally. This latter, rare condition is called 'trichophobia' (Gupta *et al*, 1990). Childhood trauma and emotional neglect may play a role in the development of this disorder (Lochner *et al*, 2002).The patients experience an increasing sense of tension immediately before an episode of hair pulling and when attempting to resist the behavior, they feel relieved of tension and sometimes a feeling of gratification after hair pulling (Enos & Plante, 2001).Trichotillomania is one of the rare conditions in which pathologic examination of the skin can be diagnostic. The hair root undergoes a unique change called trichomalacia, which only occurs in patients with trichotillomania. Thus, if the patient denies pulling his or her own hair, a skin biopsy can be helpful in determining the diagnosis. It is not always easy to convince the patient or parent that the problem is emotional rather than dermatological. At first a therapeutic relationship should be established in which the patient can be helped to accept appropriate treatment. SSRIs and clomipramine, in dosages appropriate for the treatment of obsessive-compulsive disorder, have positive treatment effects on trichotillomania. When itching is a feature, Doxepin may be the better choice. In resistant cases SSRI augmentation with pimozide, olanzapine or resperidone may be effective. The nonpharmacologic approach includes cognitive-behavior therapy with habit reversal (Keuthen *et al*, 1998).

5.3.3   Onychophagia

Onychophagia or repetitive nail biting is a common behavior that can begin as early as 4 years, with a peak between the ages of 10 and 18 years, and appears to be familial. Severe onychophagia can lead to significant medical and dental problems, such as hand infection and craniomandibular disorders. Onychotillomania, the picking or tearing of the nail, is a variant. The disorder responds to clomipramine or an SSRI. Behavioral therapy may be efficacious (Shenefelt, 2010).

5.4   Factitious Disorder and Malingering

5.4.1   Factitial dermatitis

Factitial dermatitis (dermatitis artefacta) is defined as all dermatological, self-inflicted skin lesions, where the patient denies having produced the lesions. Lesions consist of excoriations, blisters, purpura, ulcers, erythema, edema, sinuses and nodules. Methods used by patients include rubbing, scratching, picking, cutting, puncturing, sucking, biting, occlusion, application of suction cups, or dye or heat or caustic substances to the skin (Koblenzer, 2000). Skin damage can be extensive with full thickness skin loss requiring plastic surgery and even amputation. Despite the variety of skin lesions, they have some common features. Affected sites tend to be easily accessible to the patient and are more prominent on one side of the body depending on the handedness of the patient. The condition is more common in women than in men (3: 1 to 20: 1) (Gieler *et al*, 2013; Mohandas *et al*, 2013; Van Moffaert *et al*, 1985).The disorder often begins after severe psychological stress, usually involving loss, threatened loss or isolation. The most common co-morbid psychopathology is borderline personality disorder. However, some patients with borderline personality disorder readily acknowledge that they damage their skin in an impulsive act that resembles obsessive compulsive spectrum disorders and they respond to SSRIs. Other associated conditions include OCD, anxiety, depression, psychosis and mental retardation, and most of the patients with factitious dermatitis have some sort of personality disorder and they often use some means to damage his or her own skin, such as burning cigarettes, chemicals or sharp instruments (Koblenzer, 2000; Gieler *et al*, 2013; Mohandas *et al*, 2013; Van Moffaert *et al*, 1985).The management of factitious dermatitis involves the development of an empathic therapeutic relationship between the dermatologist and the patient. Because the patients deny the self-inflicted nature of the lesions, they usually do not immediately accept a referral to a psychiatrist and direct confrontation may disrupt the doctor patient relationship. However, once a therapeutic relationship has been established, some patients will accept a psychotherapeutic approach.   The prognosis varies; some cases resolve after a brief episode, whereas others become lifelong problems.

5.4.2   Munchausen's syndrome

Munchausen's syndrome is a psychiatric disorder where psychopathic behavior exists without any intention to gain something, except maybe a doctor's or nurse's attention. Skin lesions such as non-healing wounds, widespread blistering and multiple excoriations may be part of the syndrome of simulated disease. In the syndrome of Munchausen's by proxy the illness is fabricated by the parent, usually mother, or someone in loco parentis. Munchausen's by proxy can also be seen in the elderly, mentally handicapped or other dependent persons.

5.4.3   Malingering

In malingering the actions such as imitation or encouragement of illness are voluntary, with specific intention to gain something e.g. absenteeism. Cutaneous lesions are usually crude forms of artifact dermatitis. Most patients have borderline or paranoid personality disorder. Treatment is difficult and compliance erratic (Van Moffaert*et al*, 1985).

5.5   Depressive Disorders

Depressive disorders are more common in the population affected with dermatologic disorders. Comorbidity of depression and dermatologic disorders is around 30%.The correlation between depressive and dermatologic disorders still remains unclear. In depression and dermatology disorders in which certain precipitating factors are required thereby causing alteration of the patient's immunological identity causing a combination of hereditary features and ones acquired through adaptation occur to cause the disorder to develop. The cytokines are vital in the regulation of the immunology response and are also mediators of non-infective inflammatory processes leading to recurrent hormonal secretion affecting the function of the vegetative and central nervous system leading to so called "sickness behaviour", marked by loss of appetite, anhedonia, anxiety, decrease of concentration and interest along with other changes which generate a picture of depressive disorder (Filaković *et al*, 2009).

A number of investigators have found an association between skin disorders, particularly itching, and depression. The itching can be localized or generalized. Histamine, vasoactive neuropeptides and mediators of inflammation may be liberated by stress, while stress-related hemodynamic changes, variations in skin temperature and the sweat response may all contribute to existing pruritus. Scratching, a common behavioral response to stress, may compound the problem (Gupta & Gupta, 2003). A relationship of atypical pain syndromes to depressive personality structure has been hypothesized (Blumer & Heilbronn, 1984). Some cases of atypical facial pain and glossodynia fall into this category. Burning feet and possibly some cases of post-zoster neuralgia may also be included. Atypical pain syndromes are most common in women past middle life and in many cases patients exhibit a gratifying response to antidepressants. It is important to remember that steroids and antihistamines used in the treatment of skin conditions may play a role in the pathogenesis of depression and anxiety.

Depressive disease in dermatology patients can be associated with increased prevalence of suicidal ideation and substantial risk of suicide. A 5.6-7.2 % prevalence of active suicidal ideation was observed among psoriasis and acne patients which was higher than the 2.4-3.3 % prevalence of suicidal ideation observed in general medical patients (Gupta & Gupta, 2003).A substance abuse disorder such as alcohol abuse in the psoriasis patient also increases suicidal risk.

5.6   Anxiety Disorders

The physiological manifestations of anxiety disorder include increased sweating and clammy hands and feet which may present to the dermatologist. Anxiety may exacerbate disorders like psoriasis or atopic dermatitis. Having a skin disorder may induce anxiety in susceptible individuals (Shenefelt, 2010). A recent study reported that 13% of patients at a dermatology clinic had an anxiety disorder (Seyham *et al*, 2006).

5.7   Eating disorders.

Malnutrition is associated with fat tissue reduction, dry skin, purpura, petechiae, brittle hair and nails, alopecia, angular chelitis and acneform eruptions. Recidivating self-induced vomiting causes teeth enamel erosions, gingivitis and facial purpura. The skin involvement has been linked to core ego deficits and may be an index of severity in overall body image disturbance (Jaffernay, 2007; Struma, 2005).

5.8   Alcohol and Substance Abuse

Alcoholism is connected to facial erythema, teleangiectasiae, xeroderma, pruritus, urticaria, palmar erythema, cherry hemangioma, spider nevus, jaundice, hyperpigmentation and hypopigmentation. Disease states related to alcohol abuse include psoriasis, porphyria cutanea tarda, nutritional deficiencies and basal cell carcinoma (YamilaMurga *et al*, 2009). Smoking is strongly associated with numerous dermatologic conditions including poor wound healing, wrinkling and premature skin aging, squamous cell carcinoma, psoriasis, hidradenitis suppurativa, hair loss, oral cancers, and other oral conditions. In addition, it has an impact on the skin lesions observed in diabetes, lupus, and AIDS. The evidence linking smoking and melanoma, eczema, and acne is inconclusive (Freiman *et al*, 2004).Cutaneous signs of drug abuse include skin granulomas, ulcerations, recurrent infections as well as the residual scarring at the injection site (Liu *et al*, 2010).

6   Skin Disease and Sexuality

Beautiful skin is erotic and attractive and elicits a desire in the observer to touch it, while ugly skin often causes feelings of disgust, aversion and repugnance. Clinical experience shows that attention is usually paid to the sexual aspects of the skin only in venereal diseases or when the sexual organs themselves are involved. Even in such cases medical interest is concentrated on the skin lesions and less on the effects on the patient's sex life. Fifty three patients with psoriasis, 24 with atopic dermatitis and 52 controls with healthy skin were compared with regard to their sexual behavior. Patients with skin disease had significantly impaired sex lives compared to those with healthy skin. There was a highly significant reduction in the exchange of tenderness in patients of both sexes and in the capacity for orgasm in female patients, but no significant difference was found in the frequency of intercourse. Patients with psoriasis felt more impaired that those with atopic dermatitis. Ninety three percent of psoriatics and 96% of patients with atopic dermatitis had not been asked about their sexual life by their attending doctor (Niemer *et al*, 1997).

7   Management

Prior to discussing therapeutic options, it should be recognized that, if at all possible, psychodermatological cases should be referred to a psychiatrist. However, this referral process may be most optimally conducted if the dermatologist has also expressed his willingness to follow the patient with the psychiatrist so that the patient does not feel "abandoned". Although half of all prescriptions for psychotropic medications are written by nonpsychiatrists, dermatologists receive little training in prescribing such drugs (Lochner et al, 2002). However, in situations where referral to a psychiatrist is not feasible, it is within the scope of acceptable dermatological practice to try to address the psychosocial aspects of the patient's care as long as the dermatologist is knowledgeable and competent in the care given the patient. It is recognized that, within the limited setting of a dermatology practice, judicious, knowledgeable, and responsible use of psychopharmacology may be more helpful to the patient than to ignore the psychodermatology problem (Koo et al, 2003).The provision of a multidisciplinary liaison clinic within a dermatology department in a university setting may be a particularly useful way of obtaining skilled psychiatric help for the patient. The experience of some of these clinics has recently been published (Chung et al, 2012; Orion et al, 2012). The majority of patients in a Singapore Psychodermatology clinic were diagnosed with either a psychophysiologic disorder or a primary psychiatric disorder. The most common diagnosis among patients with primary psychiatric disorder was delusions of parasitosis. Other common primary psychiatric disorders seen were trichotillomania and dermatitis artefacta. About a fifth of the patients had psychiatric disorders resulting from their underlying dermatological conditions. A third of the patients were lost to follow-up. The authors conclude that managing patients with psychocutaneous disorders can be challenging, with many patients defaulting treatments. Psychodermatology clinics would benefit both patients and their caregivers. A collaborative approach using a consultation-liaison relationship between two medical departments in a friendly environment would result in more effective, integrated and holistic treatment strategies for such patients (Chung et al, 2012). During a 3-year period, 124 patients were seen in a new psychodermatology clinic in Israel, presenting with a vast array of dermatologic complaints. A major observation was that lack of proper patient-doctor communication resulted in the development of misconceptions about the disease, low compliance, and even long-lasting psychological difficulties. Another important observation was that there is a true need for such a clinic, among patients as well as among their doctors (Orion et al, 2012).

In patients with treatment-responsive skin conditions such as AD, psoriasis and acne, the issue of stress may not be important. However, when physicians are faced with disease recalcitrant to treatment, patients should be asked whether psychological, social or occupational stress might be contributing to the skin disorder. Emotional stress may exacerbate many chronic dermatoses and can initiate a vicious cycle referred to as the "itch-scratch cycle"; therefore, treatment of recalcitrant patients with chronic dermatoses may be difficult without addressing stress as an exacerbating factor.

Patients often are embarrassed about discussing psychological issues, especially if they feel hurried. Stress management classes, relaxation techniques, biofeedback, meditation, self-hypnosis, music or exercise may benefit these patients. If a specific psychosocial or occupational issue exists, therapy or counseling can help. When the patient's stress or tension is intense enough to warrant consideration of an anti-anxiety medication, two general types are available. Benzodiazepines, which can be used on an as-needed basis, provide relatively quick relief from anxiety, stress and tension. For treatment of chronic anxiety, SSRIs are safe and effective. Other options for the treatment of chronic stress include nonsedating and non-addictive anti-anxiety agents such as buspirone. If a patient's anxiety disorder warrants psychiatric referral, the referral should be discussed with the patient in a supportive and diplomatic way so that the patient is able to accept the referral as an adjunct to continuing dermatologic therapy. On the other hand, if the condition is mainly somatopsychic, this fact may provide justification to pursue a more aggressive form of treatment either by using stronger topical agents or by introducing systemic medication. Although the approach to patients may differ depending on whether the emotional distress is primarily psychosomatic or somatopsychic in nature, both types of patients can be helped by the use of anxiolytic medication (Gil et al, 1987; Gupta et al, 1989).Treatment of depressive and dermatologic disorders is complex and requires an integral therapeutic approach encompassing all aspects of both disorders and their co-morbidity. Therefore therapeutic success lies in a team approach to the patient under the auspice of consultative-liaison psychiatry by setting the frame for efficient collaboration and bridging the gap between the mental and the physical in everyday clinical practice (Filaković et al, 2009).

To summarize the following therapeutic options are available to the dermatologist or, better, can be made available through a referral.

- **Empathy**: Ensure that patients feel heard and feel that their concerns are validated Spend extra time with patients, particularly during initial diagnosis or exacerbations Enquire about the psychosocial and economic effects of skin disease.
- **Education**: Discuss the natural history, medical management, and prognosis of skin disease Dispel common misconceptions Offer an informative handout describing the condition or refer patients to support groups for psychodermatological patients.
- **Psychopharmacology**: The use of psychotropic medications requires ongoing monitoring for efficacy and side effects. If one psychotropic medication does not work adequately then it is recommended that the dose be optimized or a different agent may be tried. Commonly used medications include:
    - *Antianxiety agents*: alprazolam, buspirone, lorazepam.
    - *Antidepressants*: doxepin, fluoxetine, sertraline.
    - *Antipsychotics*: for delusions: pimozide, olanzapine, risperidone.
    - *Anti-obsessive-compulsive medications*: fluoxetine, clomipramine, paroxetine.
- **Behaviour therapy**: Behaviour therapy for patients with recalcitrant behavior disorders, such as itch-scratch cycle or chronic picking, a referral to a behaviorist may be indicated in addition to other treatment modalities.
- **Psychotherapy**: Psychotherapy is usually not feasible for a dermatologist due to lack of training and time and referral to a therapist could be useful.
- **Stress reduction**: Various methods of stress reduction such as relaxation, biofeedback, meditation, self-hypnosis, exercise, etc., can be helpful when anxiety and stress are prominent elements in the patients overall clinical picture. No specific pharmacological interventions are as yet available to prevent or treat skin disorders triggered by stress. However, based on recent advances in neuroimmunology, reasonable pharmacological treatment options are slowly emerging. Abrogation of mast-cell activation seems to be a promising approach in this endeavor, but few if any clinically available molecules can effectively inhibit mast-cell activation. Disodium cromoglycate was shown to inhibit rodent mast cells but was a very weak inhibitor of mast-cell cytokine release (Kempuraj et al, 2002). Certain flavonols, such as quercetin, are powerful inhibitors of

both prestored and newly synthesized mediators from mast cells. The combination of such flavonoids with proteoglycans, such as chondroitin sulphate, appears to provide synergistic efficacy by inhibiting both activation and secretion of mast cells (Theoharides & Bielory, 2004; Arck *et al*, 2006). Appropriate CRH-R antagonists, when available, might also provide a unique therapeutic approach in skin conditions precipitated or worsened by stress. Further, the prototypic stress-associated neuropeptide SP may be blocked by the application of a high-affinity neurokinin-1 receptor antagonist. Thus, neurokinin-1 receptor antagonists might be useful in alleviating stress-induced hair loss and skin inflammation (Arck *et al*, 2006). Apart from and in addition to the above therapeutic options, it is also important to recognize that how the dermatologist interacts with the patient has important positive (or negative) management implications (Koo *et al*, 2003).

8   Conclusion

Psychocutaneous diseases encompass a complex and diverse group of disorders. Patients with psychocutaneous disorders usually present to dermatologists for management. These patients can be particularly difficult to manage as they are often reluctant to seek psychiatric treatment. Patients may be more willing to accept a psychiatric evaluation if a psychiatrist is working within the dermatology clinic. In a study of dermatology-liaison clinic, most of the psychiatric workload involved the treatment of comorbid depressive and anxiety disorders. Furthermore, most of the patients who were seen in the liaison clinic responded well to psychiatric treatment. However, most communities do not have psychiatrists available to perform a liaison function within dermatology settings and the situation is unlikely to change in the foreseeable future (Arnold, 2005). This emphasizes the need for liaison between the specialties of psychiatry and dermatology. Such collaboration will help alleviate the suffering of many patients whose underlying illnesses may not have been otherwise clearly identified and appropriately treated.

References

Absolon, C.M., Cottrell, D., Eldridge, S.M., & Glover, M.T. (1997). Psychological disturbance in atopic eczema: the extent of the problem in school-aged children. Br J Dermatol 1997;137:241-245.

Arck, P.C., Slominski, A., Theoharides, T.C., Peters, E.M.J., & Paus, R. (2006). Neuroimmunology of Stress: Skin Takes Center Stage. Journal of Investigative Dermatology, 126(8), 1697–1704.

Arck, P., & Paus, R. (2006). From the brain-skin connection: The neuroendocrine-immune misalliance of stress and itch. Neuroimmunomodulation, 13, 347–356.

Arndt, J., Smith, N., &Tausk, F. (2008). Stress and atopic dermatitis. Current Allergy and Asthma Reports,8(4), 312-317.

Arnold, L.M. Dermatology. In Levenson, J.L. (eds) Textbook of Psychosomatic Medicine. Washington: American Psychiatric Publishing Inc. 2005. (pp 629-646).

Barankin, B., &Dekoven, J. (2002). Psychosocial effects of common skin diseases.Canadian Family Physician, 48, 712-716.

Blumer, D., & Heilbronn, M. (1984). Antidepressant Treatment for Chronic Pain Treatment Outcome of 1,000 patient's with pain-prone Disorder. Psychiatric Annals, 14, 796-800.

Bockelbrink, A., Heinrich, J., Schäfer, I., Zutavern, A., Borte, M., Herbarth, O., Schaaf, B.,von Berg, A., Schäfer, T., LISA Study Group. (2006). Atopic eczema in children: Another harmful sequel of divorce. Allergy, 61, 1397–1402.

Buske-Kirchenbaum, A., Geiben, A., Wermke, C., Pirke, K.M.,&Hellhammer, D. (2001). Preliminary evidence for herpes labialis recurrence following experimentally induced disgust. Psychotherapy & Psychosomatics, 70, 86–91.

Calikusu, C., Yücel, B., Polat, A., & Baykal, C. (2003). The relation of psychogenic excoriation with psychiatric disorders: A comparative study. Comprehensive Psychiatry, 44, 256–261.

Chaudhury, S., & Augustine, M. (1990).Monosymptomatic Hypochondriacal Psychosis. Indian Journal of Psychiatry, 32, 276-278.

Chaudhury, S., & Das, A.L. (1998a).Psychological factors in psoriasis. Indian Journal of Psychiatry, 40, 295-299.

Chaudhury, S., & Das, A.L. (1998b).Emotional factors in Alopecia areata. Medical Journal Armed Forces India, 54, 371-372.

Chaudhury, S., John, T.R., Ghosh, S.R., & Mishra, G.S. (2001).Recurrent trichobezoar in a case of trichotillomania. Indian Journal of Psychiatry, 43, 342-344.

Chaudhury, S., Raju, M.S.V.K., Salujha, S.K., Srivastava, K., &Chaudhary, A. (2003). Trichotillomania. Medical Journal Armed Forces India, 59, 65-66.

Chaudhury, S., Singh, M., & Das, A.L. (1993). Emotional factors in atopic dermatitis patients. Psychological Research Journal, 17, 15-20.

Chung, W.L., Ng, S.S., Koh, M., Peh, L.H., & Liu, T.T. (2012). A review of patients managed at a combined psychodermatology clinic: a Singapore experience. Singapore Medicine Journal, 53(12), 789-793.

Consoli, S.G. (2003). Psychologicalfactors in chronic urticaria. Annals of Dermatology&Venereology, 130, Special No.1, S73-S77.

Cotterill, J.A., &Cunliffe, W.J. (1997). Suicide in dermatologicalpatients. British Journal ofDermatology, 137, 246-250.

D'Erme, A.M., Zanieri, F., Campolmi, E., Santosuosso, U., Betti, S., Agnoletti, A.F., Cossidente, A., &Lotti, T. (2012). Therapeutic implications of adding the psychotropic drug escitalopram in the treatment of patients suffering from moderate-severe psoriasis and psychiatric comorbidity: a retrospective study. Journal of the European Academy of Dermatology and Venereology.doi: 10.1111/j.1468-3083.2012.04690.x.

Dogra, S., & Kanawar, A.J. (2002). Skin diseases: Psychological and social consequences. Indian Journal of Dermatology, 47, 197–201.

Enos, S., & Plante, T. (2001). Trichotillomania: An overview and guide to understanding. Journal of Psychosocial Nursing & Mental Health Services, 39, 10–18.

Esposito, M., Saraceno, R., Giunta, A., Maccarone, M., &Chimenti, S. (2006). An Italian study on psoriasis and depression.Dermatology, 212, 123–127.

Filaković, P., Petek, A., Koić, O., Radanović-Grgurić, L., &Degmecić, D. (2009).Comorbidity of depressive and dermatologic disorders - therapeutic aspects. Psychiatria Danubina, 21(3), 401-410.

Finlay, A.Y., & Coles, E.C. (1995). The effect of severe psoriasis on the quality of life of 369 patients. British Journal of Dermatology, 132, 236-244.

Freiman, A., Bird, G., Metelitsa, A.I., Barankin, B., &Lauzon, G.J. (2004). Cutaneous Effects of Smoking. Journal of Cutaneous Medicine & Surgery, 8, 415–423.

Garcia-Hernandez, M.J., Ruiz-Doblado, S., Rodriguez-Pichardo, A., & Camacho, F. (1999). Alopecia areata, stress and psychiatric disorders: A review. Journal of Dermatology, 26, 625–632.

Gieler, U., Consoli, S.G., Tomás-Aragones, L., Linder, D.M., Jemec, G.B., Poot, F., Szepietowski, J.C., de Korte, J., Taube, K.M., Lvov, A., &Consoli, S.M. (2013). Self-Inflicted Lesions in Dermatology: Terminology and Classification – A

Position Paper from the European Society for Dermatology and Psychiatry (ESDaP). Acta Dermatologica & Venereologica, 93(1), 4-12.

Gil, S. (2006). An overview of atopic eczema in children: a significant disease. British Journal of Nursing, 15(9), 494-499.

Gil, K. M., Keefe, F. J., Sampson, H.A., McCaskill, C.C., Rodin, J., & Crisson, J.E. (1987). The relation of stress and family environment to atopic dermatitis symptoms in children. Journal of Psychosomatic Research, 23, 673-684.

Ginsburg, I.H., & Link, B.G. (1993). Psychosocial consequences of rejection and stigma feelings in psoriasis patients. International Journal of Dermatology, 32, 587-591.

Ginsburg, I.H., & Link, B.G. (1989). Feelings of stigmatization in patients with psoriasis. Journal of the American Academy of Dermatology, 20, 53–63.

Griesemer, R.D. (1978). Emotionally triggered disease in a dermatology practice. Psychiatry Annals, 8, 49-56.

Gupta, M.A., Gupta, A.K., & Schork, N.J. (1996). Psychological factors affecting self-excoriative behavior in women with mild-to-moderate facial acne vulgaris. Psychosomatics, 37, 127-130.

Gupta, M.A., Gupta, A.K., & Schork, N.J. (1996). Psychological factors affecting self-excoriative behavior in women with mild-to-moderate facial acne vulgaris. Psychosomatics, 37, 127-130.

Gupta, M.A., & Gupta, A.K. (2003). Psychiatric and psychological co-morbidity in patients with dermatologic disorders. American Journal of Clinical Dermatology, 4, 833–842.

Gupta, M. A., Gupta, A. K., Kirkby, S., Schork, N.J., Gorr, S.K., Ellis, C.N., & Voorhees, J.J. (1989). A psychocutaneous profile of psoriasis patients who are stress reactors. General Hospital Psychiatry, 11, 166-173.

Gupta, M.A., Gupta, A.K., Schork, N.J., & Ellis, C.N. (1994). Depression modulates pruritus perception: A study of pruritus in psoriasis, atopic dermatitis, and chronic idiopathic urticaria. Psychosomatic Medicine, 56, 36–40.

Gupta, M.A., & Gupta, A.K. (2003). Depression and dermatological disorders. In Koo, J.Y.M., & Lee, C.S. (eds). Psychocutaneous medicine. New York: Marcel Dekker. (pp 233-249).

Gupta, M.A., Gupta, A.K., Ellis, C.N., & Voorhees, J.J. (1990). Some psychosomatic aspects of psoriasis.Advances in Dermatology, 5, 21–31.

Halvorsen, J.A., Stern, R.S., Dalgard, F., Thoresen, M.,Bjertness, E., &Lien, L.(2011). Suicidal ideation, mental health problems, and social impairment are increased in adolescents with acne: a population-based study. The Journal of Investigative Dermatology, 131, 363–370.

Hashizume, H., Horibe, T., Ohshima, A., Ito, T., Yagi, H., &Takigawa, M. (2005). Anxiety accelerates T-helper 2-tilted immune responses in patients with atopic dermatitis. British Journal of Dermatology, 152, 1161–1164.

Herron, M.D., Hinckley, M., Hoffman, MS., Papenfuss, J., Hansen, CB; Callis, KP., Krueger, GG. (2005). Obesity, Smoking, and Psoriasis. Archives of Dermatology, 141, 1527-1534

Jafferany, M., Vander Stoep, A., Dumitrescu A, &Hornung RL. (2010). Psychocutaneous disorders: a survey study of psychiatrists' awareness and treatment patterns. Southern Medical Journal, 103, 1199-1203.

Jafferany, M., Vander Stoep, A., Dumitrescu, A., &Hornung, R.L. (2010). The knowledge, awareness, and practice patterns of dermatologists toward psychocutaneous disorders: results of a survey study. International Journal of Dermatology, 49, 784-789.

Jaffernay, M. (2007). Psychodermatology: A guide to understanding common psychocutaneous disorders. Primary Care Companion Journal of Clinical Psychiatry, 9, 203-213.

Jowett, S., & Ryan, T. (1985). Skin disease and handicap: An Analysis of the Impact of Skin Conditions. Social Science & Medicine, 20, 425-429.

Juhlin, L. Recurrent urticaria: Clinical investigations of 330 patients. British Journal of Dermatology, 1981; 104:369–81.

Katsarou-Katsari, A., Singh, L.K., &Theoharides, T.C. (2001).Alopecia areata and affected skin CRH receptor upregulation induced by acute emotional stress.Dermatology, 203, 157–161.

Kempuraj, D., Huang, M., Kandere, K., Boucher, W., Letourneau, R., Jeudy, S., Fitzgerald, K.,Spear, K,, Athanasiou, A., &Theoharides, T.C. (2002). Azelastine is more potent than olopatadine in inhibiting interleukin-6 and tryptase release from human umbilical cord blood derived cultured mast cells. Annals of Allergy, Asthma, & Immunology, 88, 501–506.

Keuthen, N.J., O'Sullivan, R.L., &Sprich-Buckminster, S. (1998). Trichotillomania: Current issues in conceptualization and treatment. Psychotherapy & Psychosomatics, 67, 202-210.

Koblenzer, P.J. (1996).Parental issues in the treatment of chronic infantile eczema.Dermatologic Clinics, 14, 423-427.

Koblenzer, C.S. (2000). Dermatitis artefacta: clinical features and approaches to treatment. American Journal of Clinical Dermatology, 1, 47-55.

Koblenzer, C.S. (1985).Thedysmorphic syndrome. Archives of Dermatology, 121, 780–784.

Koo JYM, Lee CS, Kestenbaum T, Ginsburg, I.H., Baldwin, H., Hogarty, T., Kushon, D., Fried, R., Koblenzer, P., Koblenzer, C., Gould, W., Shephard, M.E., Cotterill, J.A. & Augustin, M. (2003). International consensus on care of psychodermatological patients.In Koo JYM, Lee CS (eds). Psychocutaneous medicine. New York: Marcel Dekker. (pp. 31-40).

Korabel, H., Dudek, D., Jaworek, A., &Wojas-Pelc, A. (2008). Psychodermatology: Psychological and psychiatrical aspects of dermatology. PrzegladLekarski, 65, 244–248.

Koshevenko, I.N. (1989). The psychological characteristics of patients with vitiligo.VestnikDermatologiiiVenerologii, 5, 4–6.

Lapidus, C.S., & Kerr, P.E. (2001). Social impact of atopic dermatitis. Medicine & Health, Rhode Island, 84, 294–295.

Lee, E. & Koo, J.Y.M. (2003). Psychiatric issues in vitiligo. In Koo, J.Y.M., & Lee, C.S. (eds). Psychocutaneous medicine. New York: Marcel Dekker (pp 351-363).

Linder, D., Dall'olio, E., Gisondi, P., Berardesca, E., Gennaro, E.D., Pennella, A.R., Giannetti, A., Peserico, A., &Girolomoni, G. (2009). Perception of disease and doctor-patient relationship experienced by patients with psoriasis: a questionnaire-based study. American Journal of Clinical Dermatology, 10(5), 325-330.

Liu, S.W.,Lien, M.H., &Fenske, N.A. (2010). The effects of alcohol and drug abuse on the skin.Clinical Dermatology, 28(4), 391-399.

Lochner, C., DuToit, P.L., Zungu-Durwayi, N., Marais, A., van Kradenburg, J., Seedat, S., Niehaus, D.J.,&Stein, D.J. (2002). Childhood trauma in obsessive- compulsive disorders, trichotillomania and controls. Depression & Anxiety, 15, 66–68.

Love, B., Byrne, C., Roberts, J., Browne, G., & Brown, B. (1987). Adult psychosocial adjustment following childhood injury: the effect of disfigurement. Journal of Burn Care & Rehabilitation, 8, 280-285.

Lowe, N.J., Glaser, D.A., Eadie, N., Daggett, S., Kowalski, J.W., & Lai, P.Y. (2007).Botulinum toxin type A in the treatment of primary axillary hyperhidrosis: A 52 week multicenter double-blind, randomized, placebo-controlled study of efficacy and safety. Journal of American Academy of Dermatology, 56, 604–611.

Mallon, E., Newton, J.N., Klassen, A., Stewart, S.L., Ryan, T.J., & Finlay, A.Y. (1999). The quality of life in acne: a comparison with general medical conditions using generic questionnaires. British Journal of Dermatology, 140: 672-676.

Mallon, E., Newton, J.N., Klassen, A., Stewart, S.L., Ryan, T.J., & Finlay, A.Y. (1999). The quality of life in acne: a comparison with general medical conditions using generic questionnaires. British Journal of Dermatology, 140: 672-676.

Mattoo, S.K., Handa, S., Kaur, I., Gupta, N., & Malhotra, R. (2001). Psychiatric morbidity in vitiligo and psoriasis: A comparative study from India. Journal of Dermatology, 28, 424–432.

Misery, L., Chastaing, M., Touboul, S., Callot, V., Schollhammer, M., Young, P., Feton-Danou, N., Dutray, S., & French Psychodermatology Group. (2012). Psychogenic skin excoriations: diagnostic criteria, semiological analysis and psychiatric profiles. ActaDermatologica&Venereologica, 92, 416-418.

Misery, L. (2011).Consequences of Psychological Distress in Adolescents with Acne.The Journal of Investigative Dermatology, 131, 290–292.

Misery, L., Feton-Danou, N., Consoli, A., Chastaing, M., Consoli, S., & Schollhammer, M. (2012).Isotretinoin and adolescent depression. Annals of Dermatology& Venereology, 139(2), 118-123.

Mohandas, P., Bewley, A., & Taylor, R. (2013). Dermatitis Artefacta and Artefactual Skin Disease: the need for a Psychodermatology Multi-Disciplinary Team to treat a difficult condition. British Journal of Dermatology. doi: 10.1111/bjd.12416.

Niemer, V., Winkelsesser, T., &Gieler, U. (1997). Skin disease and sexuality: An empirical study of sex behavior on patietns with psoriasis vulgaris and neurodermatitis in comparison with skin healthy probands. Hautarzt, 48, 629-633.

Orion, E., & Ben-Avi, O. (2011). A new psycho-dermatology clinic in Israel: our first year experience. Harefuah, 150(1), 9-12.

Orion, E., Feldman, B., Ronni, W., & Orit, B.A. (2012). A psychodermatology clinic: the concept, the format, and our observations from Israel. American Journal of Clinical Dermatol, 13(2):97-101.

Padopoulos, L., Bor, R., Legg, C., & Hawk, J.L. (1998). Impact of life events on the onset of vitiligo in adults: Preliminary evidence for a psychological dimension in etiology. Clinical & Experimental Dermatology, 23, 243–248.

Papadopoulos, L., Bor, R., & Legg, C. (1999). Coping with the disfiguring effects of vitiligo: A preliminary investigation into the effects of cognitive behavioural therapy. British Journal of Medical Psychology, 72, 385–396.

Phillips, K.A., & Dufresne, R.G. (2000).Bodydysmorphic disorder: A guide for dermatologists and cosmetic surgeons. American Journal of Clinical Dermatology,1, 235–243.

Phillips, K.A., & Dufresne, R.G. Jr. (2002). Body dysmorphic disorder: A guide for primary care physicians. Primary Care, 29, 99–111.

Picardi, A., & Abeni, D. (2001). Stressful life events and skin diseases: Disentangling evidence from myth. Psychotherapy and Psychosomatics, 70, 118–136.

Porter, J., Beuf, H., Nordlund, J.J., & Lerner, A.B. (1979). Psychological reaction to chronic skin disorders: A study of patients with vitiligo. General Hospital Psychiatry, 1, 73–77.

Porter, J., Beuf, H., Lerner, A.B., & Nordlund, J.J. (1990). The effect of vitiligo on sexual relationship. Journal of the American Academy of Dermatology, 22, 221–222.

Rapp, S.R., Feldman, S.R., Exum, M.L., Fleischer, A.B. Jr., & Reboussin, D.M. (1999). Psoriasis causes as much disability as other major medical diseases. Journal of the American Academy of Dermatology, 41, 401-407.

Rees, L. (1957). An etiological study of chronic urticaria and angioneurotic edema. Journal of Psychosomatic Research, 2, 172–189.

Russo, P.A., Ilchef, R., & Cooper, A.J. (2004). Psychiatric morbidity in psoriasis: A review. Australasian Journal of Dermatology, 45, 155–159.

Saini, R., Pande, V., Chaudhury, S., &Rathee, S.P. (2004). Body dysmorphic disorder. Industrial Psychiatry Journal, 13, 125-128.

Sampogna, F., Tabolli, S., &Abeni, D. (2007). The impact of changes in clinical severity on psychiatric morbidity in patients with psoriasis: A follow-up study. British Journal of Dermatology,57, 508–513.

Sampogna, F., Raskovic D, Guerra L, Pedicelli, C.,Tabolli, S., Leoni, L., Alessandroni, L., &Abeni, D. (2008). Identification of categories at risk for high quality of life impairment in patients with vitiligo. The British Journal of Dermatology, 159, 351–359.

Schmitt, J.M., & Ford, D.E. (2007). Role of depression in quality of life for patients with psoriasis. Dermatology, 215, 17–27.

Seyham, M., Aki, T., Karincaoglu, Y., & Ozcan, H. (2006). Psychiatric morbidity in dermatology patients: Frequency and results of consultations. Indian Journal of Dermatology, 51, 18-22.

Shenefelt, P.D. (2010). Psychological interventions in the management of common skin conditions. Psychology Research and Behavior Management, 3, 51–63.

Shiro, M., & Okumura, M. (1994). Anxiety, depression, psychosomatic symptoms and autonomic nervous function in patients with chronic urticaria. Journal of Dermatological Science, 8, 129–135.

Srinivasan, T.N., Suresh, T.R., Jayaram, V., & Fernandez, M.P. (1994). Nature and treatment of delusional parasitosis: a different experience in India. International Journal of Dermatology, 33, 851-855.

Struma, R. (2005). Dermatologic signs in patients with eating disorders. American Journal of Clinical Dermatology, 6, 165-173.

Theoharides, T.C., & Bielory L. (2004). Mast cells and mast cell mediators as targets of dietary supplements. Annals of Allergy, Asthma, & Immunology, 93(Suppl), S24–S34.

Toyoda, M., Makino, T., Kagoura, M., & Morohashi, M. (2001). Expression of neuro peptide-degrading enzymes in alopecia areata: An immunohistochemical study. British Journal of Dermatology, 144, 46–54.

Van Moffaert, M., Vermander, F., & Kint, A. (1985). Dermatitisartefacta. International Journal ofDermatology, 24, 236-238.

Willemsen, R., Roseeuw, D., & Vanderlinden, J. (2008). Alexithymia and dermatology: the state of the art. International Journal of Dermatology, 47, 903-910.

Williamson, R., Harntjens, P., Rosenow, D., & Vanderlinden, J. (2009). Alexithymia in patients with alopecia areata: Educational background much more important than traumatic events. Journal of the European Academy of Dermatology and Venereology, 23, 1141-1146.

Yadav, S., Narang, T., & Kumaran, M. S. (2013). Psychodermatology: A comprehensive review. Indian Journal of Dermatology, Venereology and Leprology, 79, 176–192.

YamilaMurga, Y., Parra, V., Aredes, A., Alasino, A., Torres, A., Santolín, L., Salomón, S., & Carena, J. (2009). Cutaneous manifestations in alcoholic patients. Relation with cirrhosis. Dermatología Argentina, 15, 77-81.

Foreign Body Reaction in the Conjunctiva and Ocular Surface Caused by Synthetic and Organic Fibers

Mohammed Kashaf Farooq
Department of Ophthalmology, Glostrup Hospital
University of Copenhagen, Denmark

Jan Ulrik Prause
Eye Pathology Institute
University of Copenhagen, Denmark

Steffen Heegaard
Department of Ophthalmology, Glostrup Hospital
Eye Pathology Institute
University of Copenhagen, Denmark

1   Introduction

Corneal and conjunctival foreign bodies generally fall under the category of minor ocular trauma. Small particles may become lodged in the corneal- or conjunctival epithelium or in the stroma, particularly when hitting the eye with considerable force.

The foreign object may set off an inflammatory cascade, resulting in dilation of the surrounding vessels and subsequent oedema of the lids, conjunctiva, and cornea. Inflammatory cells are also recruited, resulting in an anterior chamber reaction and/or corneal infiltration. If not removed, a foreign body can cause infection and/or tissue necrosis (Wilson *et al.*, 2001).

The eye can be divided into different parts that are commonly involved in immunological reactions. In this review we will be focusing upon the anterior part of the eye, which consists of the tear fluid layer, conjunctiva and cornea – the anterior ocular barrier (AOB). AOB constitutes the primary barrier against environmental aeroallergens, infectious agents and foreign bodies.

Generally, the corneal ocular foreign bodies may be grouped into 3 main categories. 1) synthetic, 2) organic and 3) metallic. In more than 70 % of the cases foreign bodies originates from metal grinding or cutting activities (Nepp *et al.*, 1999). These will just shortly be mentioned here. While the main focus of this review will be on the synthetic and organic foreign bodies. We herein describe the ocular surface defence and allergological mechanism when the AOB is exposed to foreign bodies.

2   Immunological Reaction to Foreign Body

Foreign bodies in the ocular tissue cause the formation of granuloma. Granulomas are focal, chronic, predominantly mononuclear cell driven inflammatory reactions evoked by persistent poorly biodegradable tissue irritants. The granuloma formation is either an immunological or a non-immunological (foreign body) granulomatous reaction.

Foreign body granuloma is induced by inert, non-biodegradable material. Although the cellular bulk of both types of granulomas are histiocytes and multinucleated giant cells (MGC) and their derivatives, the cell populations of granulomas differ with respect to several metabolic parameters. MGC are a common feature of both types of granuloma. MGC are highly stimulated cells of macrophage origin and are produced by cell-cell fusion induced by various cytokines, like interferon-c(IFN-c), interleukin (IL)-1, -3, -4 and -6, and granulocyte-macrophage colony stimulating factor (GM-CSF) (Hernandez *et al.*, 2000).

Some experimental studies have shown that MGC represent an adaptation for enhanced phagocytic activity and serve a useful purpose in degrading or eliminating tissue irritants that are resistant to elimination by isolated macrophages. Macrophages are found to reside in the wound and to exert long term tissue reaction. They are actively involved in removing damaged tissue and foreign body debris via phagocytosis. They release a variety of chemokines, such as interferon-γ and tumor necrosis factor-α, resulting in an enhanced microbial or tumoricidal capacity and release of pro-inflammatory cytokines and cell mediators (Hernandez *et al.*, 2000, Su *et al.*, 2011).

The above mentioned granuloma formation is also taking place in the conjunctiva, that is a well vascularized tissue that contains large numbers of dendritic/Langerhans cells and macrophages (Kari & Saari, 2012). This is different in the cornea. The anatomy of the cornea is optimized for transparency in order to allow maximal light transmission. The cornea consists mainly of a relatively dense connective tissue (stroma) built up by tightly arranged lamellae of collagen bundles. The cornea contains relatively few cells in the stroma, and these are so-called keratocytes (modified fibrocytes). There are no lymphoid cells or other apparent protective elements, apart from some dendritic cells and their precursors. For a number of functions such as moistening and nutrition, and also for the purpose of defence, the cornea therefore depends largely on its major support tissue – the conjunctiva (Knop & Knop, 2005). For this reason granuloma formation in the cornea only occurs after a prolonged period of untreated infection/inflammation, when there is vessel formation in the cornea (Papadopoulos *et al.*, 1998).

3   Foreign Bodies

Superficial foreign bodies in the cornea cause discomfort rather than acute pain. When the deeper part of the cornea is involved pain is normally more intense, and the patient may not be able to cooperate until the pain is relieved. Establishing the velocity of the foreign body at the impact is essential. Low velocity foreign bodies will normally be found in the conjunctiva, the subtarsal plate or on the cornea. High velocity foreign bodies can enter the globe or the orbit (Jones, 1998).

Metallic foreign bodies account for the majority of foreign bodies found on the cornea and in the conjunctiva, but a wide variety of different aetiological foreign bodies have been described in the literature. These can generally be divided into synthetic and organic foreign bodies, ranging from pieces of wood or insect wings to synthetic fibers from a teddy bear or polyethylene foreign bodies (Covert *et al.*, 2009, Fogla *et al.*, 2001, Bansal *et al.*, 2008).

3.1   Metallic

In more than 70 % of the cases foreign bodies originates from metal grinding or cutting activities. Superficial corneal foreign bodies are one of the leading causes of ocular trauma, affecting mainly young males who work with metal under strain, as locksmiths, mechanics and stoneworkers (Nepp *et al.*, 1999, Koray *et al.*, 2007). One of the most common reasons of metallic foreign bodies is welding-related injury. The welding process may expose workers to various sources of mechanical, radiant, thermal, or chemical energy (Pabley & Keeney, 1981). Often the foreign body is superficial but if introduced to the eye with considerable velocity it may cause more serious ocular complications, such as traumatic cataract, iris or pupillary deformities, and retinal detachment. Furthermore, posttraumatic endophthalmitis is one of the most severe complications of ocular trauma because of its poor prognosis. It is recommended to perform an orbital computed tomography, if an intra- ocular or -orbital foreign body is suspected (Davidson & Sivalingam, 2002).

3.2   Organic

Different types of organic corneal foreign bodies have been described in the literature. These may include wood and insect wing bodies (Covert *et al.*, 2009, Fogla *et al.*, 2001, Portero *et al.*, 2013). We will focus on caterpillar hair and tarantula hair foreign bodies of the AOB in the following.

3.2.1   Caterpillar

Caterpillars are the larval form of members of the order *Lepidoptera* (the insect order comprising butter-flies and moths). These insects fall victim to many larger predators, and have therefor developed irritating hairs, sharp spines, and various toxins as defense mechanisms (Hossler, 2010).

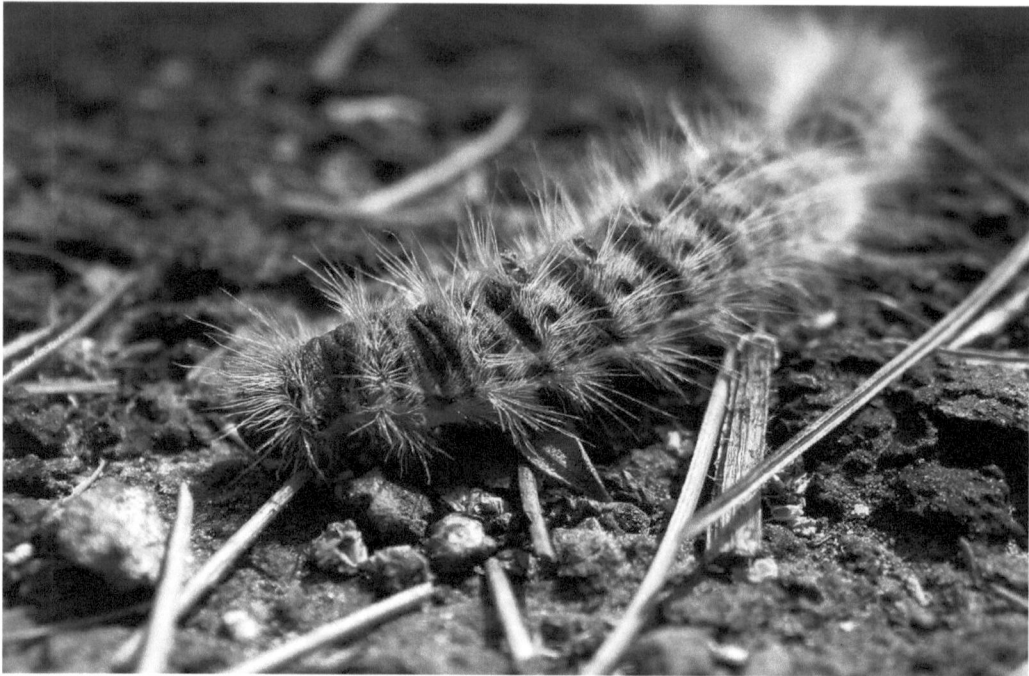

Figure 1: Larva of pine processionary *(Thaumetopoea pityocampa)*.

Contact with the hairs can cause skin rashes. The caterpillar hairs can produce an acute IgE-mediated contact urticaria, especially on the body extremities. Moreover, the embedded hairs can induce delayed cutaneous reactions that produce small infiltrated papules, papulo-vesicles, or pustules due to a toxic irritant mechanism that is not mediated by IgE (Vega *et al.*, 2003, Vega *et al.,* 1999).

The ophthalmological symptoms can also be separated into immediate IgE-dependent and delayed hypersensitivity processes. The IgE-mediated process generally produces red eye, punctate keratitis, and itchiness of the ocular surface. The delayed corneal reactions are produced as a response to the embedded caterpillar hairs. The reaction appears as stromal granulomas around the hairs days after contact (Sengupta *et al.*, 2010, Portero *et al.*, 2013). The later reaction is known as "opthalmia nodosa" and was first described by Saemisch in 1904 (Watson & Sevel, 1966). The term describes granulomatous nodules in the conjunctiva and iris due to caterpillar sensory setae. In 1966 one of the first case series was published in Europe and the different degrees of orbital involvement described (Watson & Sevel, 1966).

In 1984 Cadera *et al.* classified the ocular inflammatory manifestations in the following different clinical entities (Cadera *et al.*, 1984).

- Type I: An acute, anaphylactoid reaction to the hair, starting immediately and lasting a few days, causing chemosis and inflammation.

- Type II: Chronic mechanical kerato conjunctivitis caused by hair lodged in the bulbar or palpebral conjunctiva, leading to linear corneal abrasions.

- Type III: Formation of grayish-yellow granulomatous nodules in the conjunctiva. The hair may be subconjunctival or intracorneal and may be asymptomatic.

- Type IV: Iritis secondary to hair penetration into the anterior segment. The iritis may be very severe with iris nodule formation and even a hypopyon.

- Type V: Vitreoretinal involvement after hair penetration into the posterior segment.

The pathophysiologic mechanisms of these reactions are poorly understood but may involve irritant reactions, hypersensitivity reactions, and toxic envenomation (Hossler, 2010). An initially acute inflammation is followed by a granulomatous reaction around the hair. This is characterized by a lymphocytic infiltration, which is later followed by histiocytes presenting as epitheloid cells and giant cells. The lids, conjunctival fornices, subconjunctival space, cornea, and iris are most commonly involved. In the more severe reactions there is a perivascular infiltration of inflammatory cells in the retina, extending into the scleral channels and the episcleral tissues (Watson & Sevel, 1966).

From a larger subcontinental retrospective analysis, the majority of the cases were limited to manifestations of the above-mentioned type I to type III reactions (Sengupta *et al.*, 2010). Recently a smaller European case series showed keratitis as the most common ocular presentation of embedded hairs from the caterpillar (Portero *et al.*, 2013).

The prognosis is relatively good even with intraocular penetration of the hair. Despite the severe range of the manifestations, the outcome in most of the cases is satisfactory, if diagnosed early and treated appropriately. The superficially located hairs should be removed. The removal of the deeper located hairs could do more harm than good and should be clinically closely observed (Horng *et al.*, 2000, Conrath *et al.*, 2000, Corkey, 1955). The application of steroid ointments is recommended. Anti-allergic medication may provide relief from periocular edema or skin urticating lesions. The condition tends to be self-resolving over a period of weeks or months, with symptoms becoming reduced over time. The presence of intracorneal hair is a significant risk factor for intraocular penetration (Sengupta *et al.*, 2010, Horng *et al.*, 2000, Conrath *et al.*, 2000).

3.2.2   Tarantula Hairs

Tarantulas are becoming an increasingly popular choice as pets. Some of them are relatively small, affordable and widely available at pet stores. While many of these pet tarantulas are considered relatively safe due to their lack of poison or fangs, they pose a non-realized danger from their defensive hairs (Rutzen *et al.*, 1993, Battisti *et al.*, 2011). These urticating hairs or setae are released easily from the abdomen with mechanical stimulation. If provoked, the tarantula will discharge a spray of setae by rapidly vibrating both hind legs as a defence mechanism (Battisti *et al.*, 2011). Both caterpillar sensory setae and the urticating hairs of the tarantula are pointed and barbed and the tendency to cause ocular inflammation seems to be similar (Hered *et al.*, 1988, Cadera *et al.*, 1984).

Four types of hairs have been classified and range from 0.06 mm to 1.5 mm in size. Type 3 hairs, are supposed to penetrate the skin and ocular surface and cause irritation (Cooke *et al.*, 1972). The irritant effect is thought to be primarily mechanical, while the role of a toxin or hypersensitivity reaction is not fully understood.

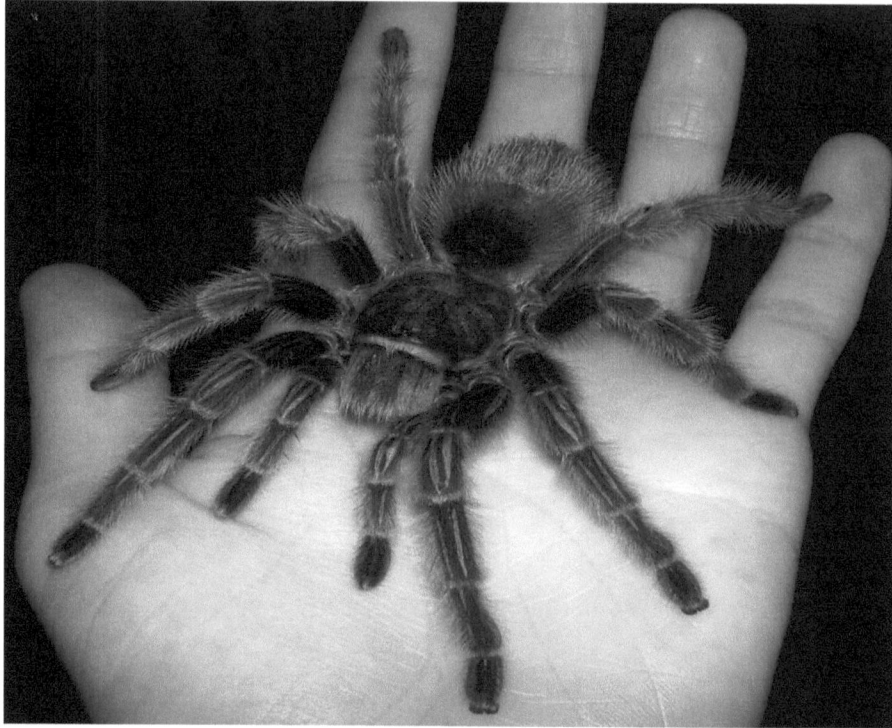

Figure 2: *Chilian Rose Hair Tarantula.*

Tarantula hairs have been reported to cause a number of medical ocular conditions in humans (Mangat & Newman, 2012, Watts *et al.*, 2000, Waggoner & Nishimoto, 1997, Hered *et al.*, 1988). It has been shown that the hairs can penetrate the corneal tissue with either the barbed or the smooth end (Kaufman *et al.*, 1994). Though it has been proposed that the hairs inflict injury initially through an acute inflammatory reaction followed by chronic granulomatous inflammation, there is also evidence that the hairs penetrate the ocular tissues apparently without inciting inflammation or causing fibrosis (Kaufman *et al.*, 1994, Bansal *et al.*, 2008). Specific lesions such as the focal damage and loss of corneal endothelial cells have also been visualized using the confocal microscope in rabbits (Kaufman *et al.*, 1994).

The insect setae consist of a chitin skeleton with a matrix of proteins and covered by layers of lip-oproteins, mucopolysaccharides and other constituents. These are foreign to mammals and may act as a strong inducer of inflammation and potentiator of mammals' immune responses. Chitin particles can bind to receptors on macrophages and activate them to produce chitinases together with proinflammatory cy-tokines and other inflammatory and immune regulatory mediators (Battisti *et al.*, 2011).

The initial symptom and clinical manifestations are skin urticarial or conjunctival hyperemia. This may be followed by a chronic granulomatous type reaction, resulting in nodular conjunctivitis, stromal keratitis, mutton-fat keratitic precipitates, iritis, vitritis, and multifocal punctate chorioretinal lesions (Mangat & Newman, 2012, Watts *et al.*, 2000, Shrum *et al.*, 1999).

Hered *et al.* recommends removal of offending hairs, or at least close observation of their move-ment to determine if surgical removal is necessary (Hered *et al.*, 1988). Another study advocates the use of confocal microscopy for optimal diagnosis and follow up (Kaufman *et al.*, 1994). Ocular injury from the barbed hairs of tarantulas is of particular concern due to the popularity of tarantulas as household.

3.3   Synthetic

Synthetic fibers from stuffed toy animals and blankets made of synthetic material may penetrate the conjunctiva or cornea. This may result from close exposure of stuffed toy animals to the eye (Weinberg *et al.*, 1984, Schmack *et al.*, 2005). Usually as mentioned earlier, the foreign bodies are removed from the ocular surface by the eye protective mechanisms such as blinking and tearing. However, foreign bodies may be retained and encapsulated by the mucous and initiate a local inflammatory response (Mantelli & Argüeso, 2008, Zierhut & Stiemer, 1997, Adams, 1976). This may, in the conjunctiva, give rise to granuloma formation, also known as "Teddy bear granuloma", first described by Weinberg *et al.* in 1984.

   We will be presenting two unique cases of synthetic foreign body granuloma formation in conjunctival epithelium and in cornea, respectively. These cases have been published formerly (Farooq *et al.*, 2011).

3.3.1   Case 1

A 2-year-old girl presented with ocular irritation and corneal opacities of her left eye. Topical treatment with ciprofloxacin and chloramphenicol for suspected conjunctivitis had no improvement on the condition. No trauma or any foreign body complaints was observed or recalled according to the patient's mother. Apart from mild asthma the patient was in a healthy medical condition.

   Examination in general anaesthesia revealed a 4 x 5 mm oval ulceration infero-centrally of the left cornea with purulent exudate, stromal oedema and a couple of large "mutton fat" precipitates.

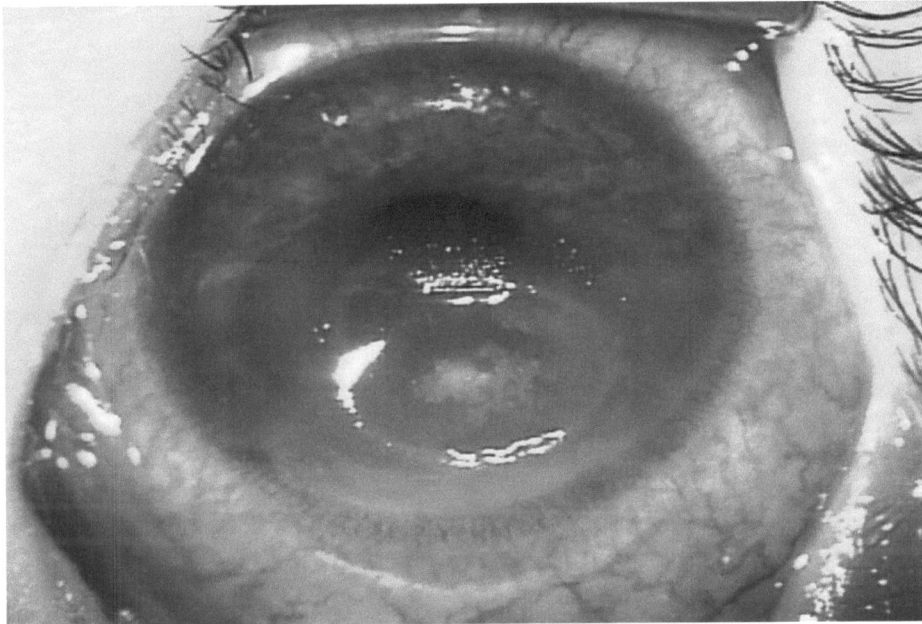

Figure 3: Corneal ulceration measuring 4x5 mm

   No foreign bodies were detected. In addition a severe iritis with synechiae and a hypopyon less than one mm was found. Conjunctival and corneal swabs were sent for bacterial and fungal staining and culture. Due to a clinically suspected bacterial infection, topical treatment was changed to oxytetracyclinpolymyxin-B ointment, ciprofloxacin and chloramphenicol eye drops six times daily and topical atropine once daily.

For the next two weeks there was a remarkable improvement of the corneal ulceration. However, suddenly a relapse with a new hypopyon and worsening of the corneal ulceration occurred. The treatment was supplemented with fortified gentamicin and fortified cefuroxin eye drops every hour. One week later the results of the staining and the cultures were proved negative for bacteria and fungi. The condition worsened and a spontaneous perforation occurred centrally in the ulceration. Furthermore, a new but smaller ulceration was observed more laterally. Corneal transplantation was performed and the corneal button was sent for microscopical examination. The results from the light microscopy showed a heavily inflamed and ulcerated cornea.

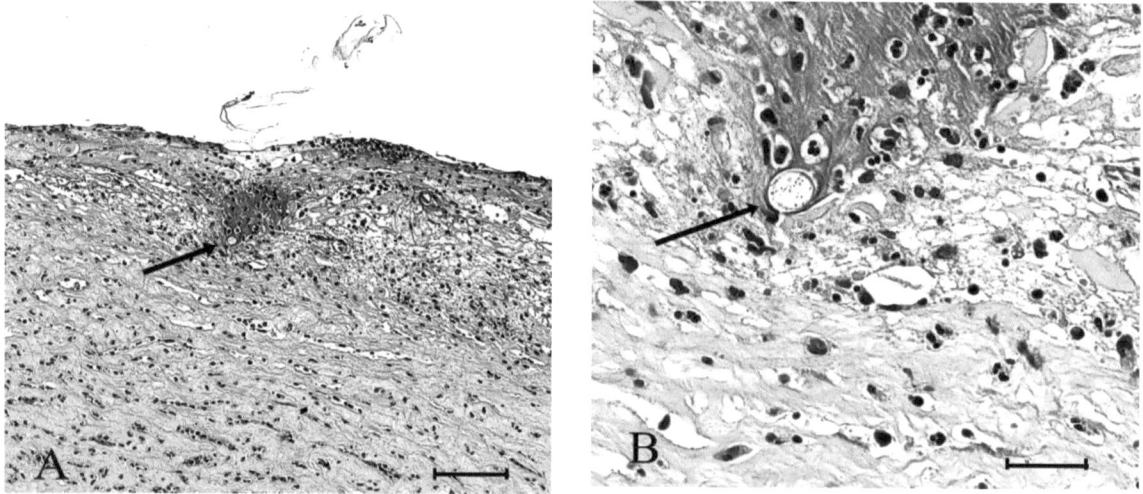

Figure 4: Haematoxylin-eosin (HE) staining of the inflamed corneal biopsy. The stroma contains multiple histiocytes and neutrophils and is embedded with bluish brown synthetic fibers (arrows) exhibiting central black granular spots. Bars: 150 μm (A), 50 μm (B).

Bowman's layer was missing and the ulceration occupied most of the stroma reaching Descement's membrane. The stroma contained a granulomatous lesion with multiple histiocytes and neutrophils. Numerous rounds to oval shaped blue and brown fibers with black granular spots were seen centrally in the lesion. The diameter of the fibers ranged from 20-30 μm and showed strong birefringence in polarized light (figure 4).

To verify whether the synthetic fibers belonged to a toy teddy bear, we performed microscopical examination of two different types of synthetic fibers (whiskers and face hair) from the girl's toy teddy bear (figure 5). Hairs from the face were morphologically and microscopically identical with the fibers causing the severe corneal ulceration in the two-year-old girl.

Investigation of the teddy bear fur demonstrated that the fiber was made of 100% polyethylene (Dacron, Terylene). The azo-dye (Faron Dark Blue, Clariant), applied to the fibers is not restricted by EU and is not known to cause inflammation.

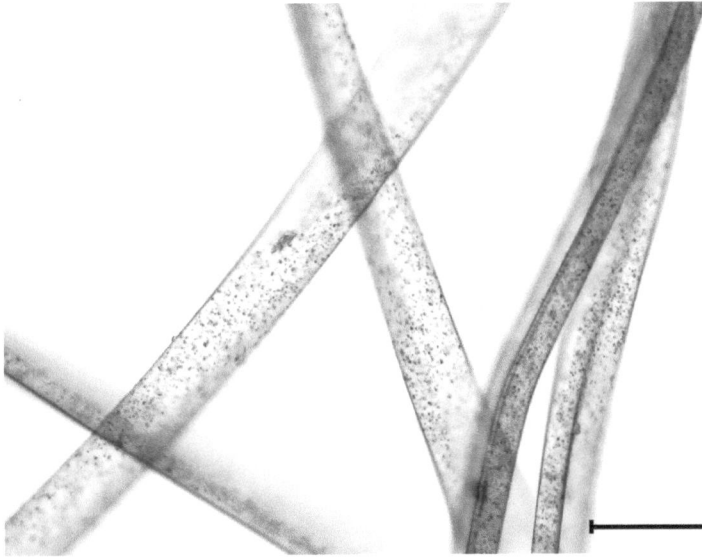

Figure 5: Light microscopy of teddy bear hair. Bar: 50 μm.

3.3.2   Case 2

A five-year-old girl was admitted to the eye department because of irritation and foreign body sensation in her left eye for two days. She was otherwise in a good general health.

Slit lamp examination showed a 7 x 5 mm granuloma in the left inferior conjunctival fornix embedded with hairs and synthetic fibers. The lesion prolapsed easily with gentle pressure on the left lower lid. The examination was otherwise normal. The lesion was excised under general anaesthesia and sent for microscopical examination. Postoperatively, the eye was treated with chloramphenicol three times daily for five days. The wound healed within two weeks and the postoperative course was uneventful.

Microscopical examination of the conjunctiva revealed a normal differentiated conjunctival epithelium with goblet cells. The subepithelial stroma contained a granuloma with inflammatory cells, mostly eosinophils, histiocytes and foreign body giant cells. Synthetic fibers, identified by their strong birefringence in polarized light were found within the lesion (Figure 6). The diameter of the fibers ranged from 20-30 μm. We could not identify the chemical composition of these fibers.

3.3.3   Comments

Increased tear flow, redness, foreign body sensation, pain and photophobia are the symptoms associated with foreign body in the eye. Signs of possible deeper ocular penetration include decreased vision and clouding of the cornea (Lueder, 1999). However, the symptoms expressed by children or the toddler may be nonspecific, as they might be unable to communicate properly.

The majority of the previously described patients with conjunctival granuloma (caused by synthetic foreign bodies) were referred to an eye department after the granuloma was visible (Schmack *et al.*, 2005). This may in children take weeks since children may neglect the symptoms until the granuloma has developed, or because the symptoms communicated to the parents are misunderstood (Schmack *et al.*, 2005, McGrath, 1990). However, in the present case of conjunctival granuloma signs were seen early and the child was referred after two days.

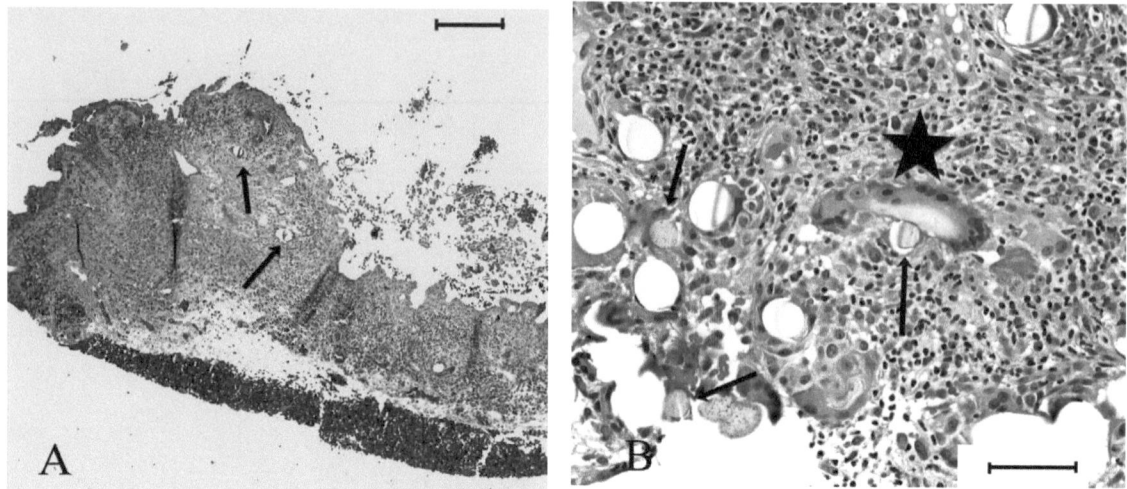

Figure 6: HE stained conjunctival biopsy. The connective tissue is infiltrated with inflammatory cells mostly eosinophils, and synthetic fibers (black arrows) surrounded by foreign body giant cell (asterisk). Bars: 200 µm (A), 50 µm (B).

Even though the patient with the corneal ulceration was examined with slit lamp, the examiner was unable to identify the corneal foreign body. A main reason might be that the synthetic fibers were bluish brown, similar to the colour of hypopyon and the iris. Thus causing difficulties identifying the foreign body. However, a careful slit lamp examination combined with a negative bacterial and fungal staining and culturing should lead to the proper diagnosis.

Tarantula hairs and caterpillar setae foreign bodies in the eye are well documented (Watson, 1966, Cadera *et al.*, 1984, Hered *et al.*, 1988). However, so far only this present case of synthetic fiber causing severe ocular complications is reported in the literature (Farooq *et al.*, 2011). The lesions are considered partly due to penetration and partly to the inflammatory/toxic reaction, in the same way as hairs from the tarantula back are supposed to cause irritation to the skin (Cooke *et al.*, 1973). Whether the same mechanisms are responsible for the severe case of keratitis in our case is unclear. However, it is plausible that the synthetic fibers may cause an allergic and toxic reaction in the cornea. The synthetic fibers in case one were made of polyethylene. When used in joint arthroplasty, polyethylene may cause an osteolytic reaction when small particles are engulfed by macrophages in granulomatous reactions (Heisel *et al.*, 2004). The azo dye applied in the fibers may also have had an influence; however, it has not been documented to have any adverse effect.

In 2005 Schmack *et al.* demonstrated the histopathological and ultrastructural features of conjunctival granulomas caused by synthetic fibers. The diagnosis is easily confirmed by the microscopical features of the conjunctival granuloma showing granulomatous inflammatory tissue with lymphocytes, plasma cells, eosinophils and usually foreign-body giant cells surrounding the synthetic fibers. The simplest method to confirm the diagnosis is excision of the conjunctival granuloma end microscopical examination demonstrating marked birefringence of the synthetic fiber when examined in polarized light (Enzenauer & Speers, 2002, Resnick *et al.*, 1991). The synthetic fibers are fairly uniform in diameter and generally round to oval in configuration. The diameter of synthetic fibers in the cases published by Schmack *et al.* and Weinberg *et al.* ranged from 17-29 µm and 21-27 µm, respectively, which is also suggested in our case (Schmack *et al.*, 2005, Weinberg *et al.*, 1984). The localization of the granuloma in the previously published 15 cases was unilateral and mainly in the inferior fornix, except in one case in the superior fornix (Schmack *et al.*, 2005).

The ocular surface epithelium not only acts as a physical and mechanical barrier against harmful substances, but also participates actively during allergic inflammatory processes (Calonge *et al.*, 2005). Patients with asthma might react with a profound ocular hypersensitivity (Hesselmar *et al*, 2010). Thus, the formation of a corneal granuloma, in the patient with known asthma (case 1) could have been potentiated by local ocular allergic reactions.

Surgical removal of the conjunctival granuloma and postoperative treatment with antibiotics is recommended and has shown to be successful (Enzenauer & Speers, 2002, Lueder *et al*, 1996). The crucial element in the treatment of keratitis is the identification of the cause of the keratitis. In young children rare causes such as synthetic fibers should always be kept in mind, especially in children who are attached to their toy teddy bears. Identification and removal of the corneal and conjunctival foreign body granuloma followed by antibiotic administration are the treatment of choice.

References

Adams DO. (1976). *The granulomatous inflammatory response, a review. Am J Pathol. 84(1), 164-192.*

Bansal R, Ramasubramanian A. Jain AK, Sanghi G. (2008). *Polyethylene foreign body on the cornea. Cornea. 27(5), 605-8.*

Battisti A, Holm G, Fagrell B, Larsson S. (2011). *Urticating hairs in arthropods: their nature and medical significance. Annu Rev Entomol. 56, 203–220.*

Cadera W, Pachtman MA, Fountain JA, Ellis FD, Wilson FM. (1984). *Ocular lesions caused by caterpillar hairs. Can J Ophthalmol. 19(1), 40-4.*

Calonge M & Enríquez-de-Salamanca A (2005). *The role of the conjunctival epithelium in ocular allergy. Curr Opin Allergy Clin Immunol. 5(5), 441-445.*

Conrath J, Hadjadj E, Balansard B, Ridings B. (2000). *Caterpillar setae-induced acute anterior uveitis: a case report. Am J Ophthalmol. 130(6), 841-3.*

Cooke J, Roth V, Vincent D, Miller F (1972), *The urticating hairs of theraphosid spiders. Am Museum Noviates 2498, 1-43.*

Cooke JA, Miller FH, Grover RW, Duffy JL (1973). *Urticaria caused by tarantula hairs. Am J Trop Med Hyg 22(1), 130-133.*

Corkey JA. (1955). *Ophthalmia nodosa due to caterpillar hairs. Br J Ophthalmol. 39(5), 301–306.*

Covert DJ, Henry CR. Shelth BP. (2009). *Well-tolerated intracorneal wood foreign body of 40-year duration. Cornea. 28(5), 597-8.*

Davidson RS & Sivalingam A. (2002). *A metallic foreign body presenting in the anterior chamber angle. CLAO J. 28(1), 9–11.*

Enzenauer RW & Speers WC (2002). *Teddy bear granuloma of the conjunctiva. J Pediatr Ophthalmol Strabismus. 39(1), 46-48.*

Farooq MK, Prause JJ, Heegaard S. (2011). *Synthetic fiber from a teddy bear causing keratitis and conjunctival granuloma: case report. BMC Ophthalmology. 20, 11:17.*

Figure 1: http://commons.wikimedia.org/wiki/File:Thaumetopoea_pityocampa_larva.jpg

Figure 2: http://commons.wikimedia.org/wiki/File:Grammostola_rosea_Chilian_Rose_Hair_Tarantula.jpg

Fogla R, Rao SK, Anand AR, Madhavan HN. (2001). Insect Wing Case: Unusual Foreign Body. Cornea 20(1), 119–121.

Heisel C, Silva M, Schmalzried TP (2004). Bearing Surface Options for Total Hip Replacement in Young Patients. Instr Course Lect. 53, 49-65.

Hered RW, Spaulding AG, Sanitato JJ, Wander AH. (1988). Ophthalmia nodosa caused by tarantula hairs. Ophthalmology. 95(2), 166-169.

Hernandez-Pando R, Bornstein QL, Aguilar LD, Orozco EH, Madrigal VK, Martinez CE. (2000). Inflammatory cytokine production by immunological and foreign body multinucleated giant cells. Immunology. 100(3), 352-8.

Hesselmar B, Bergin AM, Park H, Hahn-Zoric M, Eriksson B, Hanson LA, Padyukov L (2010). Interleukin-4 receptor polymorphisms in asthma and allergy: relation to different disease phenotypes. Acta Paediatr. 99(3), 399-403.

Horng CT, Chou PI, Liang JB. (2000). Caterpillar setae in the deep cornea and anterior chamber. Am J Ophthalmol. 129(3), 384-5.

Hossler EW. (2010). Caterpillars and moths. Part I. Dermatologic manifestations of encounters with Lepidoptera. J Am Acad Dermatology. 62(1), 1-10.

Jones G. (1998). Foreign bodies in the eye. Accid Emerg Nurs. 6(2), 66-9.

Kari O & Saari KM. (2012). Diagnostics and new developments in the treatment of ocular allergies. Curr Allergy Asthma Rep. 12(3), 232-9.

Kaufman SC, Chew SJ, Capps SC, Beuerman RW.Scanning. (1994). Confocal microscopy of corneal penetration by tarantula hairs. Scanning. 16(5), 312-5.

Knop E & Knop N. (2005). The role of eye-associated lymphoid tissue in corneal immune protection. J Anat. 206(3), 271-85.

Koray G, Sarper K, Mirza E. (2007). Case Report. Corneal Injury From a Metallic Foreign Body: An Occupational Hazard. Eye & Contact Lens 33(5), 259–260.

Lueder GT. (1999). Synthetic granuloma. Arch Fam Med. 8(5), 376-377.

Lueder GT, Matsumoto B, Smith ME (1996). Pathological case of the month. Synthetic fiber granuloma ("teddy bear granuloma"). Arch Pediatr Adolesc Med. 150(3), 327-328.

Mangat SS & Newman B. (2012). Tarantula hair keratitis. N Z Med J. 125(1364), 107-10.

Mantelli F & Argüeso P. (2008). Functions of ocular surface mucins in health and disease. Curr Opin Allergy Clin I munol. 8(5), 477-483.

McGrath PA, 1 ed. (1990). Pain in children – Nature, assessment and treatment. New York: Guilford Press.

Nepp J, Rainer G, Krepler K, Stolba U, Wedrich A. (1999). Etiology of non-penetrating corneal injuries. Klin Monatsabl Augenheilkd. 215(6), 334-7.

Pabley AS & Keeney AH. (1981). Welding processes and ocular hazards and protection. Am J Ophthalmol. 92(1), 77–84.

Papadopoulos M, Snibson GR, McKelvie PA. (1998). Pyogenic granuloma of the cornea Australian and New Zealand Journal of Ogbtbcllmology. Aust N Z J Ophthalmol. 26(2), 185-88.

Portero A, Carreno E, Galarreta D, Herreras JM. (2013). Corneal Inflammation from Pine Processionary Caterpillar Hairs. Cornea. 32(2), 161-4.

Schmack I, Kang SJ, Grossniklaus HE, Lambert SR. (2005). Conjunctival granulomas caused by synthetic fibers: Report of two cases and review of literature. J AAPOS. 9(6), 567-571.

Sengupta S, Reddy PR, Gyatsho J, Ravindran RD, Thiruvengadakrishnan K, Vaidee V. (2010). Risk factors for intraocular penetration of caterpillar hair in Ophthalmia Nodosa: a retrospective analysis. Indian J Ophthalmol. 58(6), 540-3.

Resnick SC, Schainker BA, Ortiz JM (1991). Conjunctival synthetic and nonsynthetic fiber granulomas. Cornea. 10(1), 59-62.

Rutzen AR, Weiss JS, Kachadoorian H. (1993). Tarantula hair ophthalmia nodosa. Am J Ophthalmol. 116(3), 381– 382.

Shrum KR, Robertson DM, Baratz KH, Casperson TJ, Rostvold JA. (1999). Keratitis and retinitis secondary to tarantula hair. Arch Ophthalmol. 117(8), 1096-7.

Su J, Todorov M, Gonzales HP, Perkins L, Kojouharov H, Weng H, Tang L. (2011). A Predictive Tool for Foreign Body Fibrotic Reactions Using 2-dimensional computational model. Open Access Bioinformatics. 2011(3), 19-35.

Vega ML, Vega J, Vega JM, Moneo I, Sanchez E, Miranda A. (2003). Cutaneous reactions to pine processionary caterpillar (Thaumetopoea pityocampa) in pediatric population. Pediatr Allergy Immunol. 14(6), 482–486.

Vega JM, Moneo I, Armentia A, Fernandez A, Vega J, Sanchis ME. (1999). Allergy to the pine processionary caterpillar (Thaumetopoea pityocampa). Clin Exp Allergy. 29(10), 1418–1423.

Watson P. G. & Sevel D. (1966). Ophthalmia nodosa. Br J Ophthalmol. 50(4), 209–217.

Watts P, Mcpherson R, Hawksworth NR. (2000). Tarantula keratouveitis. Cornea. 19(3), 393-4.

Waggoner TL, Nishimoto JH, Eng J. (1997). Eye injury from tarantula. J Am Optom Assoc. 68(3),188-90.

Weinberg JC, Eagle RC, Font RL, Streeten BW, Hidayat A, Morris DA. (1984). Conjunctival synthetic fiber granuloma: a lesion that resembles conjunctivitis nodosa. Ophthalmology. 91(7), 867-872.

Wilson SE, Mohan RR, Ambrosio R, Hong J, Lee J. (2001). The Corneal Wound Healing Response - Cytokine-mediated Interaction of the Epithelium, Stroma, and Inflammatory Cells. Progress in Retinal and Eye, 20(5), 625–637.

Zierhut M & Stiemer R. (1997). Physiological protective mechanisms of the eye. Klin Monbl Augenheilkd. 211(1), 1-11.

Podoconiosis: Tropical Lymphedema of the Lower Legs

Fasil Tekola-Ayele
Center for Research on Genomics and Global Health
National Human Genome Research Institute
National Institutes of Health, USA

Wendemagegn Enbiale Yeshanehe
Human Resource Development and Management
Federal Ministry of Health, Ethiopia

1   Introduction

Podoconiosis is a non-infectious, familial, geochemical lymphedema of the lower legs (Figure 1). It affects subsistence farmers in tropical highland parts of Africa and is caused by long-term barefoot exposure to red clay soil of volcanic origin (Price, 1990; Davey et al., 2007). The story of elephantiasis goes as far back as the second millennium BC. For a long period of time all forms of elephantiasis were considered infectious by most scholars until 1924 when Robles reported endemic non-filarial elephantiasis of the lower legs and described the risk factors, geographical distribution, and clinical presentations based on his study in Guatemala. Later in the 1960s and 1970s, Oomen and Price did seminal work in the epidemiology, etiology, pathology, natural history and management of non-filarial elephantiasis in Ethiopia (Oomen, 1969a; Price, 1976a; Price & Henderson, 1978). Price coined the term podoconiosis for non-filarial elephantiasis to distinguish it from filarial elephantiasis. The term was derived from the Greek terms *podos* and *konos*, which mean foot and dust, respectively and imply that the disease is caused by exposure of feet to irritant clay soil (Davey et al., 2007). The next sections of this chapter describe the epidemiology, genetics, pathogenesis, clinical presentation, diagnosis, treatment, prevention, and elimination of podoconiosis.

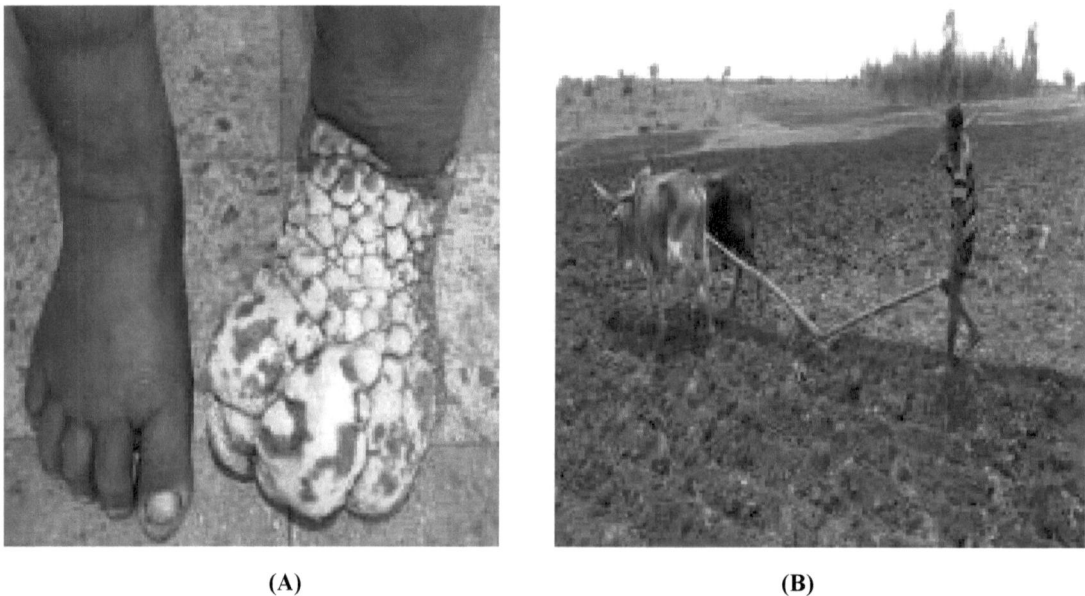

(A)   (B)

Figure 1: Podoconiosis. (A) Nodular form of podoconiosis of an adult patient in North Ethiopia.
(B) A 14 year old barefoot man plowing farming land in a podoconiosis endemic village.

2   Epidemiology

Globally, it is estimated that there are at least four million people with podoconiosis. The disease has been reported in more than 20 countries, of which ten had high burden of the disease. Countries where podoconiosis is common are mainly found in tropical Africa, central and south America and northern India (Figure 2) (Davey *et al.*, 2007). Yet recognition of the worldwide distribution of the disease has been delayed by many factors, and unlike filarial elephantiasis it is not reported in medical statistics.

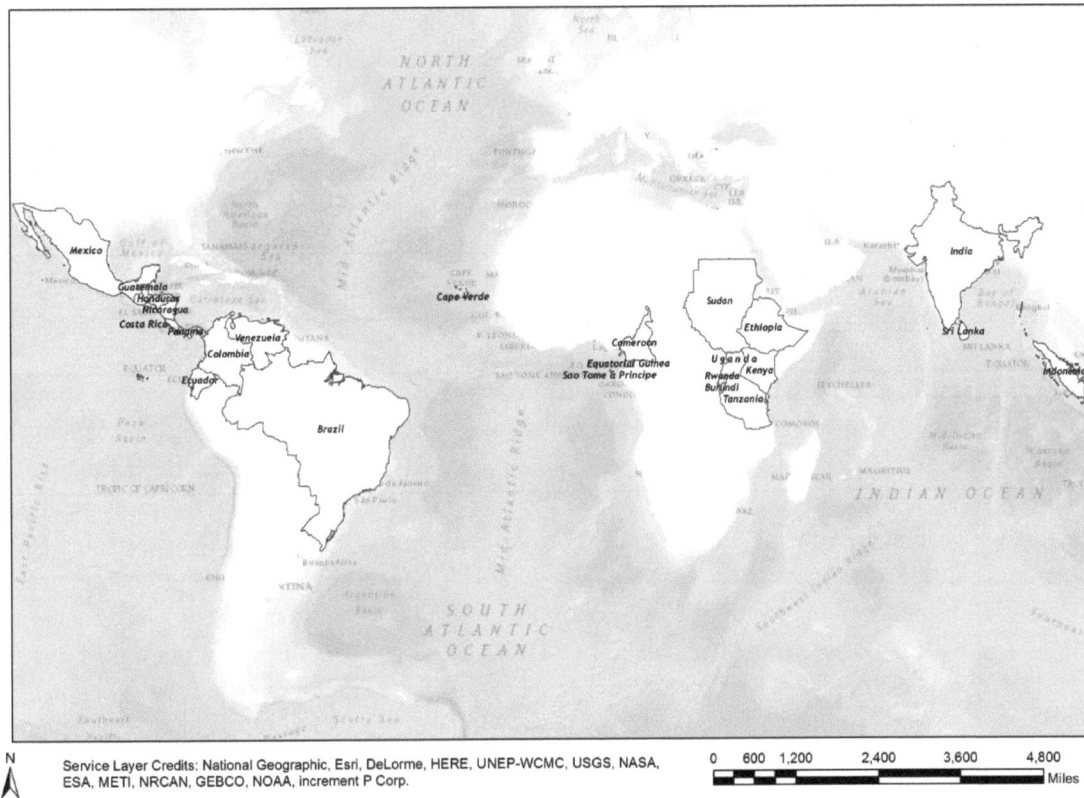

Figure 2: Geographical distribution of countries in which podoconiosis is endemic or has been described.

Podoconiosis is mostly common among agricultural people who work barefoot, particularly on red clay soils of volcanic areas (Price & Henderson, 1981; Price *et al.*, 1981; Price, 1990; Destas *et al.*, 2003). The distribution of podoconiosis shows correlation with the distribution of red clay soil derived from volcanic rocks. This association between tropical red clay soil and the occurrence of podoconiosis has been tested and shown in the East African regions of Kenya, north western Tanzania, Ethiopia, and Rwanda (Price, 1976b). Affected areas have altitude over 1000 meters, annual rainfall above 1000mm, average temperatures of ~20°C (all of which govern the type of soil produced), and soils of volcanic origin (Price, 1990).

In endemic highland areas of these countries podoconiosis is more prevalent than commonly known diseases such as HIV/AIDS, tuberculosis, malaria, or filarial elephantiasis. Ethiopia, with an estimated 1 million podoconiosis patients, has the largest number of podoconiosis patients reported so far. Studies over the past ten years have documented that the prevalence of podoconiosis ranges from 2.8% to 7.4 % in endemic areas of Ethiopia (Kloos *et al.*, 1992; Destas *et al.*, 2003; Alemu *et al.*, 2011; Geshere Oli *et al.*, 2012; Molla *et al.*, 2012a; Molla *et al.* 2012b). However, podoconiosis has not yet been adequately incorporated in the health management and information systems, health professionals' education curricula, and governmental health facility services.

Podoconiosis is more common among barefoot farmers that are exposed to currently unknown antigens in red clay soils of highland areas. Inorganic particles in red clay soils derived from volcanic rocks are considered to be the putative risk or causal factors that trigger the inflammatory process. In addition, the majority of podoconiosis patients are poor and uneducated, consequently unable to afford protective shoes or unaware of the role of wearing shoes and washing feet to prevent development of the disease (Davey *et al.*, 2007). The average age of onset of podoconiosis is in the second and third decades of life (Destas *et al.*, 2003; Alemu *et al.*, 2011; Molla *et al.*, 2012b). Studies in different parts of Ethiopia have documented different patterns of burden of podoconiosis in men and women. Some studies have shown that men and women are equally affected, others have shown that the disease disproportionately affects women than men, and a third group of studies have found that the gender ratio varies by the severity of the disease with more men affected at the late stages of podoconiosis (Kloos *et al.*, 1992; Destas *et al.*, 2003; Alemu *et al.*, 2011; Geshere Oli *et al.*, 2012; Molla *et al.*, 2012b).

Besides the high prevalence of podoconiosis in endemic areas, it also imposes immense physical, social and economic burden on affected communities (Yakob *et al.*, 2008; Tekola *et al.*, 2009; Yakob *et al.*, 2010; Tora *et al.*, 2011). Most patients experience recurrent bacterial and fungal super infection of the lower leg leading to loss of productivity. Almost all patients have five or more episodes of acute lymphadenitis per year, and on average loss one month of an annual economic activity because of morbidity (Alemu *et al.*, 2011; Molla *et al.*, 2012a; Molla *et al.*, 2012b). An estimation of the economic costs of podoconiosis in southern Ethiopia has shown that in an area with 1.7 million residents, the annual economic cost of podoconiosis is more than 16 million USD per year, costing Ethiopia more than 200 million USD. Comparison of affected and unaffected people employed with the same job shows that individuals with podoconiosis are half as productive as those without. In addition, podoconiosis patients loss 45% of their economically productive time because of morbidity associated with the disease (Tekola *et al.*, 2006). About 25% of patients have diminished ability to participate in economically productive work, and some resort to begging in bigger cities (Kloos *et al.*, 1992; Molla *et al.*, 2012b). Podoconiosis is also known to have catastrophic social burden in disease endemic communities. In endemic areas podoconiosis is one of the commonest causes of stigmatization against community members. The main reasons for prevailing discrimination against patients and affected families are the erroneous belief that the disease cannot be prevented, treated or controlled; association of the disease with curses; and the belief that the disease runs in families through hereditary factors that are inevitable. Once a diseased individual is identified in a family lineage (bloodline), the whole family becomes subjected to social stigma and discrimination. Consequently, young women have meager prospects for marriage; adult patients are excluded from public gatherings such as religious places, social meetings, and public transportation facilities because of bad odor of oozing discharge; and children with podoconiosis are discriminated by peers and teachers and drop out of school. Because of such wide scale and severe stigmatization, patients also undergo self-stigmatization and isolate themselves from unaffected community members; hide their swollen legs; and hesitate to seek treatment at health facilities. Even worse, misconceptions about the cause of podoconiosis and discriminatory attitudes and practices are also exhibited by the majority of health professionals that work in disease endemic areas (Yakob *et al.*, 2008; Yakob *et al.*, 2010; Tora *et al.*, 2011).

3   Familial Clustering and Genetics

Familial aggregation of podoconiosis has been reported through expert observations, epidemiological studies, and pedigree analyses. Observations in Ethiopia and Rwanda showed that several households have more than one affected member (Price, 1972b; Price, 1976b). In addition, recently, studies in north and west Ethiopia have shown that reportedly one-third to half of patients have other affected close relatives (Alemu *et al.*, 2011; Molla *et al.*, 2012b). Price conducted a pedigree study in Ethiopia and for the first time, indicated that there is a genetic component in podoconiosis susceptibility with 15-40% risk genotype frequency (Price ,1972b). After a gap of more than two decades, in 2005 a pedigree study was conducted in Ethiopia using multiply affected and multi-generational families. The results showed that the genetic basis of podoconiosis is strong. The sibling recurrence risk ratio was 5.07 (i.e., the sibling of an affected person is at five times increased risk of developing podoconiosis when compared to a person in the general population); the heritability of podoconiosis was estimated to be 0.629 (i.e., 63% of the variation in development of podoconiosis is accounted for by genetic factors); and the most parsimonious model revealed the contributions of a major gene, and the roles of age, and history of use of footwear as environmental covariates (Davey *et al.*, 2007). In 2012 a genome-wide association study involving population-based podoconiosis cases and unaffected controls from southern Ethiopia revealed that genetic variants in the HLA locus of chromosome 6 confer susceptibility to podoconiosis. Specifically, single nucleotide polymorphisms in or near the class II HLA genes namely *HLA-DQA1*, *HLA-DRB1*, and *HLA-DQB1* were found to be at significantly higher frequency among podoconiosis cases than controls recruited from the same area and population group. The study findings were further corroborated with family-based association test and high resolution sequence-based HLA typing, suggest that podoconiosis is a T-cell mediated inflammatory condition (Tekola Ayele *et al.*, 2012a). Further studies to discern the causal genetic variants, the immunologic and pathologic mechanisms are underway.

4   Clinical Presentation

The clinical picture and course of podoconiosis vary based on time of presentation (early and late) and type of the lymphedema (water bag versus sclerotic or both) (Price, 1990) (Figure 3).

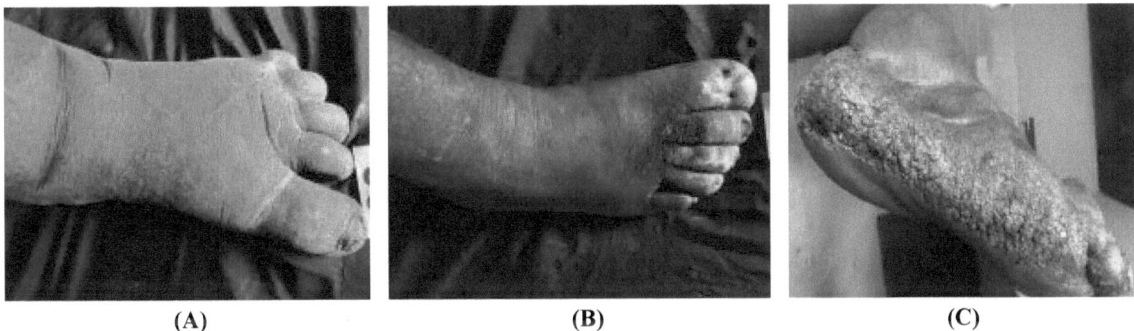

(A)   **(B)**   **(C)**

Figure 3: (A) Early edema of the foot with splaying of the big toe. **(B)** Lichenification on the dorsum of the anterior foot. **(C)** Mossy growth on the lateral part of the foot in slippery distribution.

4.1   Early Symptoms

The main presentation of the patient early on the course can be burning sensation or/and itching on the foot. The burning foot is characterized by patients, as on and off burning sensation on the foot following a day-long barefoot exposure on the farm or field. Occasionally, the patient may associate the condition with traditional beer consumption or for females with menstruation. Sometimes the burning pain may extend into the lower leg and be associated with fever and a tender femoral lymph node. In most patients this may continue for several years affecting one limb. Onset in the other limb may not occur for many months or years. Each episode of attacks resolves spontaneously or after a few days of rest and elevation of the affected limb. The itching on foot is described by the patient as persistent or intermittent itching of the dorsum of the foot, often over the dorsum of the anterior one third and in the first or second web space. Constant rubbing leads to a reactive thickening of the skin (lichenification) suggesting chronic eczema. Repetitive scratching may lead to a breach in barrier function of the skin, which may lead to recurrent cellulites or lymphangitis (Barreiro et al., 2008).

4.2   Early Signs

Identification of the earliest signs of podoconiosis is helpful for timely intervention which will have the potential to halt progression of the disease. The three key early signs are (i) Leg swelling – a transient edema of the lower leg specially the foot which increases following long working day and disappears in the morning after overnight rest (leg elevation). At this stage the edema can be pitting. The unilateral foot edema can be associated with pitting on the anterior foot pad and splaying of the forefoot, widening of the forefoot with separation of the toe, particularly between the first and the second toes. The swelling of the forefoot may cause the toes to lack their usual curvature, appearing as sausages. The deep edema of the plantar foot may lift the toe off the ground (Figure 3A). (ii) Thickening of the skin – the skin over the anterior and dorsum one third of the foot becomes lichenified and thickening can occur which renders the skin (Figure 3B), particularly overlying the first toe web space, stiff and unable to be pinched (positive Stemmer's sign). The increased skin markings, usually longitudinal, may be evident and exaggerated by squeezing together the toes; it is significantly visible between the first and second toes. (iii) Mossy foot – warty and papilomatous growth with rough surface are usually seen on the foot involving the dorsum of foot in the anterior one third and the sole of foot in slippery distribution accentuating lateral side of sole and the heel of foot. This hyperkeratotic and wart growth looks like a 'moss' but it is rough to touch (Figure 3C). Patients who have started to wear shoes usually do not have the hyperkeratotic lesion. A mismatched and asymmetric enlargement of the second toe on the affected foot is a common finding (Price, 1990).

4.3   Later Symptoms

Following the recurrent burning episodes associated with transient swelling, the leg diameter progressively increases and establishes a persistent lymphedema. The late clinical picture can vary greatly. Conventionally, three main forms of lymphedema are distinguished in podoconiosis: (1) Soft and pitting ("water bag" type) – subdermal edema that is soft to the touch and pits with pressure; it has little dermal fibrosis. Usually the swelling has a narrow neck around the knee and wider base on the foot. The skin will have a smooth and dumpy surface, with occasional lymphorhea especially on the foot which attracts flies. Often there is loss of normal hair. With time, the foot and lower leg become large and flabby (Figure 4A). With elevation there is considerable reduction in size. Swelling may lead to redundant skin folds around the ankle joint and ballooning over the toes. The disability to the patient is due to the great size of the limb and heaviness. (2) Hard and sclerotic/fibrotic or leathery leg 'elephantiasis' – sclerosis governs the changes in the skin and sub cutis, which become woody hard and grossly thickened. The overlying epidermis on the foot takes on a sandpaper-like appearance which eventually, due to increasing hyperkeratosis, takes on the so-called 'mossy' appearance (Figure 4B).

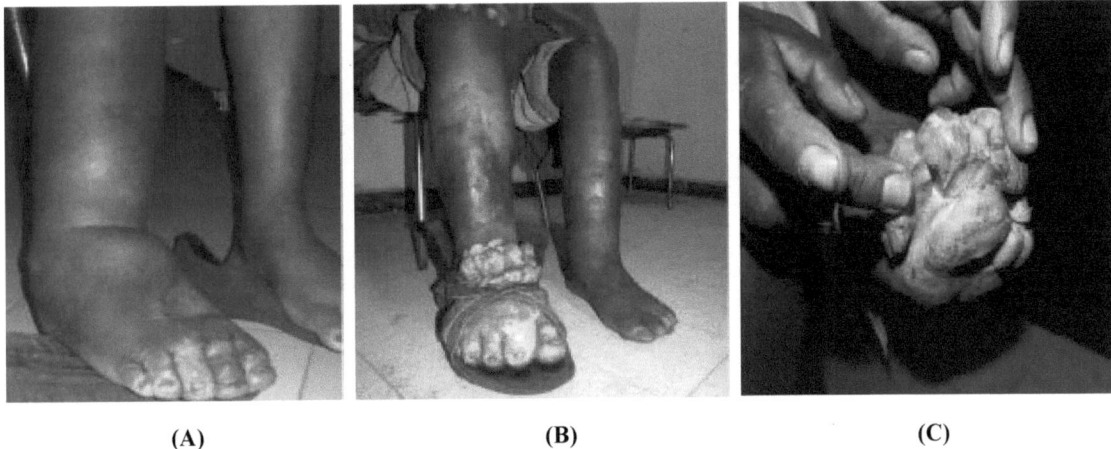

(A)   (B)   (C)

Figure 4: (A) Water bag pitting. **(B)** Fibrotic swelling with nodularity. **(C)** Oozing and macera-tion on skin folds.

Under areas of compression, such as a sandal strap, the skin remains smooth and dumpy. The stiff, sclerotic nature of this altered skin especially on the ankle compromises the normal flexibility of the ankle and toe which makes it vulnerable to cracking and trauma, in addition to ankylosis of the joints. (3) Mixed elephantiasis – characterized by grossly swollen limb below the knee and non-pitting edema, not reducible overnight (leg elevation) and no sclerotic change. There may be variation in the compressibility between the lymphedema below the ankle and above the ankle.

4.4   Other Clinical Features Associated with Podoconiosis

(1) Fibrous nodules– these lumps of redundant skin with subepidermal fibrosis occur mostly on the dorsum of the toe and foot (Figure 4B). They tend to occur mostly with the fibrotic (sclerotic) and the mixed lymphedema. The nodules can start as smooth surface skin folds and progress to timorous growth which considerably inhibits footwear.

(2) Inter-digital and skin fold maceration– whitish and wet patches on the interdigital space with occasional fissuring. The maceration is associated with oozing (lymphorhea) and usually has bacterial and fungal infections. Dumpy foot from the lymphorhea with microbial super-infection leads to the foul smell which adds to the stigma and social isolation of the patient (Figure 4C).

(3) Acute lymphangio adenitis (ALA) or cellulites– in general lymphedematous limb is said to have compromised immunologic clearance mechanism which leads to recurrent infection. One of the commonest causes of morbidity in podoconiosis is ALA affecting about 97% patients (Alemu *et al.*, 2011) with a recurrence rate of 5 to 5.5 times per year and in each attack the patient becomes bedridden for 4 days. ALA manifests as acute pain on the limb with fever, chills and rigor. The limb becomes reddened, hot and tender with tender swelling in the draining femoral lymph node (Alemu *et al.*, 2011; Molla *et al.*, 2012b).

(4) Fusions of toes– some podoconiosis patients present with toe fusions which starts on the fourth and second inter-digital spaces forming a web-like skin growth connecting the toe from proximal and extending distally (Price, 1990).

(5) Scaring and de-pigmentation– recurrent itching and ulcerative skin on the dorsum of foot results in scarring and de-pigmentation of the skin on the distal foot. The scarring causes toe resorption which confuses with leprosy (Price, 1990; Davey et al., 2007; Barreiro et al., 2008).

5   Pathogenesis

The etiology of podoconiosis has not yet been completely understood. Based on existing evidence the most accepted cause of podoconiosis is inorganic particle induced inflammatory response on a background of genetic susceptibility (Davey et al., 2007). Mineral particles, absorbed through the skin of the foot, are taken up into macrophages in the lower limb lymphatics and induce an inflammatory response in the lymphatic vessels, leading to fibrosis and obstruction of the vessel lumen. This leads initially to edema of the foot and the lower leg, which progresses to elephantiasis: gross lymphedema with mossy and nodular changes of the skin (Price, 1976a).

The historical account of studies conducted to identify the etiology of podoconiosis goes back to the 1960s. A possible etiology was suggested by Heather and Price on observing inorganic silica particles in section of femoral lymph node. A study by Price and Pitwell about the mineral content of the lymph nodes in barefoot people with and without elephantiasis of the legs confirmed presence of elements including silicon, aluminum, and iron in all barefoot people, with slightly higher amount in those with elephantiasis suggesting the etiological significance of these particles (Price & Henderson, 1978). In addition, endemic areas were free of filariasis; footwear had a protective effect; birefringent silica particles were found in the lymph node macrophages; and the dermal content of various mineral elements was consistent with local soils, leading to the postulation of soil induced disease (Price, 1972a; Price, 1976a; Price, 1990). After he conducted epidemiological and geological studies, Price indicated that silicate particles cause subendothelial edema, endolymphangitis, collagenisation and obliteration of the lymphatic lumen (Price, 1976a). Biopsies from inguinal and femoral lymph nodes of affected individuals have shown the presence of birefringent particles and foreign body granuloma (Price, 1972a). Electron microscopy of the lymph node biopsy and micro-analysis showed that the particles are found inside the macrophages and consist dominantly silica with varying amount of aluminum, titanium and iron oxide (Price & Henderson, 1978).

Histopathological examination of the lymph nodes showed that they contained birefringent minerals which, by microanalysis, were identified as sub-micron particles of kaolinite and small amounts of quartz, hematite, geothite and gibbsite (Abrahams, 2002). When crystalline silica was injected into lymphatic vessels in the legs of rabbits, it resulted in macrophage proliferation followed by lymphatic fibrosis and blockage similar to that seen in podoconiosis (Fyfe & Price, 1985). Price hypothesized that individual differences in the tissue handling of absorbed minerals plays a role in development of full-blown podoconiosis (Price, 1990). It is probable that certain minerals reach the nodes by transit through the afferent lymphatics after being absorbed through the plantar skin. Because of the known fibrogenic potency of silica, the hypothesis has emerged that the disease is an obstructive lymphopathy caused by fibrotic response to silica of soil origin. Animal study of injecting silica particles has shown that the obstructive effect of silica within the lymphatic system is on the lymphatics themselves and not on the draining lymph nodes (Price et al., 1981).

Histological examination of the lymphedematous skin shows epidermal hyperkeratosis, acanthosis and hypergranulosis (Figure 5).

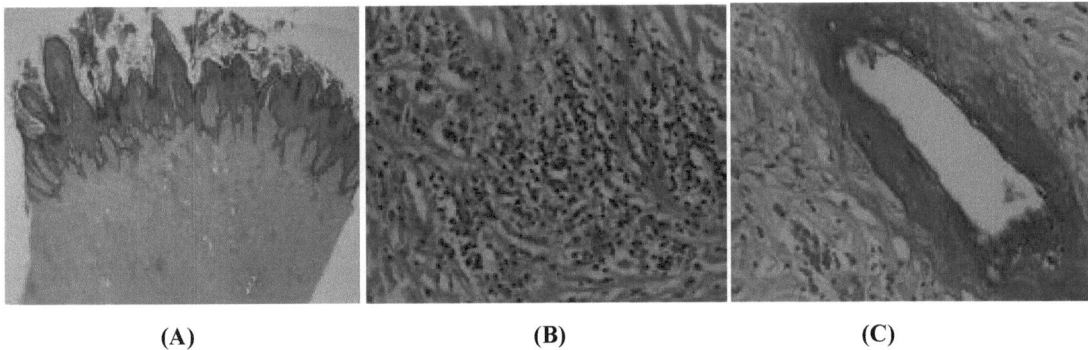

(A)   (B)   (C)

Figure 5: Histology of podoconiosis (courtesy of Almut Böer-Auer, MD, PhD, Dermatologikum, Hamburg, Germany) **(A)** H & E staining showing hyperkeratosis, acanthosis, thick whirly collagen. **(B)** H & E staining showing cellular infiltrates of lymphocyte, mast cells and plasma cells. **(C)** Collagen IV stain showing dilated blood vessels with surrounding fibrosis.

This may be a consequence of growth factors released by the inflammatory cells, which are attracted to the irritant. The papillary dermis shows fibrosis and a perivascular infiltrate of lymphocytes, mast cells, and plasma cells plus coarse, wiry bundles of collagen. The deeper dermis shows sclerosis, reflecting temporal progression of the fibrosis. The presence of dilated blood vessels with surrounding fibrosis mimics the findings of stasis. But, there are no hemosiderin deposits. This feature, together with dermal sclerosis, contributes to the hardness and irreversibility of lesions.

A recent study in northern Ethiopia has indicated that patients with podoconiosis have significantly lower stratum corneum hydration in the skin of their lower legs and feet than unaffected individuals from the same community, suggesting increased risk of cracking, susceptibility to infection, and lymphedema (Ferguson *et al.*, 2013). By comparing cases of podoconiosis at early and advanced disease stage and unaffected controls from the same area, a study has found differences in serum levels of oxidative stress biomarker levels and TGFβ1, suggesting their role in pathogenesis of podoconiosis (Addisu *et al.*, 2010).

6   Diagnosis

In endemic areas, the diagnosis of podoconiosis is usually made clinically by enquiring the history of illness and pattern of progression of the swelling, physical examination of the swollen sites, exclusion of other causes of lymphedema, and sometimes family history of the disease. At presentation, patients characterize the illness as burning sensation of the foot followed by an upwards progressive swelling that starts from the foot or lower legs and progresses upwards to the level of the knees and a gradual increase in leg circumference (Price, 1990).

The commonest differential diagnoses of podoconiosis are filarial elephantiasis, lymphedema of systemic disease and leprotic lymphoedema. In podoconiosis, the foot is the site of first symptoms (which occur elsewhere in the leg in filarial elephantiasis); the swelling is bilateral, asymmetric, usually below the level of the knees, and rarely involves the groin, whereas in filarial disease, it is predominantly unilateral and extends above the knee; sensory perception of the peripheral nerves is intact in the toes and forefoot, neurotrophic ulcers and thickened neurovascular nerves are lacking, and there is no hand involvement (unlike leprotic lymphoedema) (Price, 1990; Davey *et al.*, 2007). Earlier studies, between 1935 and 1940, of numerous cases of elephantiasis in Shoa, the then central province of Ethiopia, revealed no microfilariae in the peripheral blood taken either by day or by night. Similarly, no microfilariae were detected in 50 cases of elephantiasis examined in the Harar province, Eastern Ethiopia (Cohen, 1960; Oomen, 1969a). Likewise, onchocerciasis and lymphatic filariasis were not reported in a mission hospital in Wolaita zone, southern Ethiopia for more than 30 years, which made the presence of *Wuchereria bancrofti* unlikely (Oomen, 1969b). Recently, a study using both midnight thick film examination and Binax[TM] antigen cards has excluded filariasis as the cause of podoconiosis in Wolaita zone (Desta *et al.*, 2007). A study in central Ethiopia has also shown absence of *W. bancrofti* in the serum of individuals diagnosed with podoconiosis by lay and shortly trained community health workers (Geshere Oli *et al.*, 2012). Endemic Kaposi's sarcoma and podoconiosis share common features, such as involvement of the lymphatic system in barefoot farmers, and high prevalence in volcanic areas. This may suggest a common pathogenesis. However, they do not seem to co-exist in endemic areas (Ziegler, 1993; Ziegler *et al.*, 2001; Nenoff *et al.*, 2009). A recent study has assessed the extent to which podoconiosis can be accurately diagnosed by community health workers' clinical examination in comparison with a 'gold standard' rapid filarial antigen testing using Binax antigen cards. The study found that clinical examination of patients with podoconiosis in endemic communities has a strong predictive value to exclude filarial elephantiasis, and a valid means for diagnosing podoconiosis (Desta *et al.*, 2007).

Diagnosis of podoconiosis is often delayed because of the erroneous belief that podoconiosis can neither be treated or controlled, the prevailing stigmatization against patients when they disclose their illness, and health professionals' confusion of podoconiosis with filarial elephantiasis (Yakob *et al.*, 2010). As a consequence, active treatment seeking by patients at modern health facilities is poor. Mobilization of patients and case tracing through house-to-house surveys was the most prominent practice to encourage patients to seek care at facilities that provide such services (Davey & Burridge, 2009).

7   Treatment and Prognosis

The conventional therapy in a poor setting is composed of five components:

(1) Foot hygiene — patients will be advised to wash their feet daily in an antiseptic solution for 10 to 15 minutes and rinse it with clean water (Figure 6A).

(2) Application of emollient and massaging the skin of the affected limb.

(3) Elevation of the foot above the hip whilst resting, at least at night but also as often as is practical during the day.

(4) Compression therapy with short stretchable bandage — patient will be trained on bandaging technique. The bandage will be applied throughout the day except on the bathing time. If this is not possible, some compression can be achieved with the wearing of long socks (Figure 6B).

(5) Footwear — custom made shoes are advised where possible until the foot is of a size where more generic shoes can fit. This is to provide protection of the foot from the irritant soil as well as supporting compression (Figure 6C).

Early stages of podoconiosis lymphedema can be reversed and those with water bag type of lymphedema will have a control compatible to normal socio-economic position. Patients with woody hard fibrous nodules (Figure 3) on the foot and leg tend not to respond to this conventional therapy since the nodules are too hard to be reduced by compression bandaging.

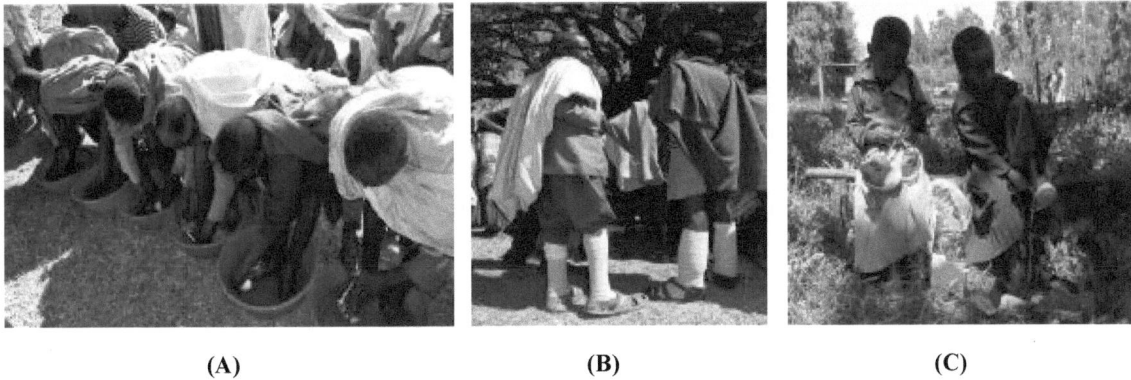

Figure 6: Treatment and prevention of podoconiosis. **(A)** Washing. **(B)** Bandaging. **(C)** Shoe wearing from childhood as prevention method.

Removal of the nodules in these patients allows them to use custom designed shoes and to control disease progress with the conventional simple management plan described above. However, any surgical intervention in patients with lymphoedema has its risks. Wound healing is known to be impaired in the context of lymphoedema so surgical intervention is advised to be undertaken with caution. Surgical excision of the nodules (nodulectomy) has been practiced in Ethiopia and we have demonstrated that surgical nodulectomies can be performed with satisfactory healing rates, encouraging lack of complications and leading to significant improvement in quality of life in a tropical low income setting (Figure 7).

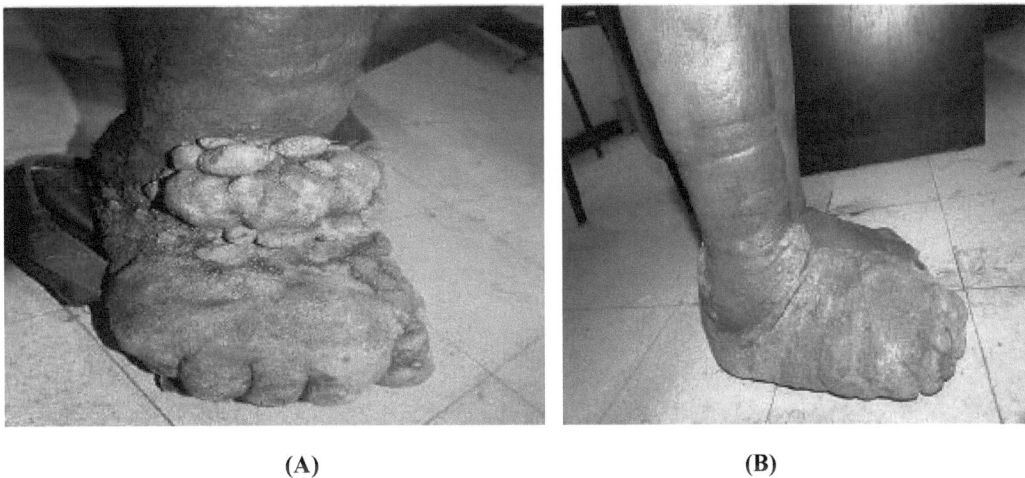

Figure 7: Surgical excision of nodules (nodulectomy) in an adult podoconiosis patient from northern Ethiopia. **(A)** Before nodulectomy. **(B)** After nodulectomy.

Treatment outcome and prognosis is monitored with indicators such as reduction of leg circumference, improvement of skin texture, clinical stage of the disease, and rate of wound healing (if they have). A one year follow-up of podoconiosis patients in Southern Ethiopia has shown dramatic improvement in the quality of life of patients (Sikorski *et al.*, 2010).

8   Prevention and Elimination

Podoconiosis is a preventable disease. Existing evidence indicates that effective prevention of podoconiosis can be achieved by regularly wearing shoes and washing feet from childhood. In early onset disease, foot hygiene is very helpful to halt and reverse progress. It involves washing feet with soap and water, use of antiseptic and emollients, and consistently wearing shoes and socks. Treatment of early stages of podoconiosis helps improve the quality of life of patients as demonstrated in a Dermatology Life Quality Index (DLQI) measurement study (Henok & Davey, 2008). In endemic areas a gradual rise in shoe wearing has been reported. For example, in north and west Ethiopia 76% and 91% of podoconiosis patients approached for surveys conducted in 2010 and 2011 were observed to be wearing shoes (Alemu et al., 2011; Molla et al., 2012). Discounting the more rigorous use of footwear among patients after the disease develops, it can be estimated that a large majority of community members have started wearing shoes. These figures are higher than those reported two to three decades ago (Kloos et al., 1992). However, financial barriers have still impacted the ability of individuals to afford better quality and more number of shoes per year (Klimentidis et al., 2011). Whether the shoes worn by the communities provide sufficient protection against the irritant particles in the soil and the consistency of usage of shoes needs thorough investigation. In addition, podoconiosis is getting a relatively better attention by global health advocates and local health institutional management bureaus. These elements can be harnessed to increase resources available for health education on personal hygiene and for improving access to shoes and water.

In addition to being a preventable disease, podoconiosis can also be eliminated from a country or an endemic area. The experience of countries such as Ireland, France, the Canary Islands that had podoconiosis in the past but have no cases currently gives hope that with universal use of foot wear and proper personal hygiene elimination of podoconiosis from endemic countries is within reach. In 2007 the Mossy Foot Treatment and Prevention Association (MFTPA) in southern Ethiopia has developed and implemented a strategy that aimed to prevent podoconiosis by targeting resources such as shoes to children who are from families with history of podoconiosis. Family history of podoconiosis captures genetic, socio-economic and behavioral risk factors shared among family members. Using this approach, the MFTPA has distributed over 40,000 pairs of shoes to children at high risk for podoconiosis (Tekola Ayele et al., 2012b). Scaling up this strategy throughout endemic areas can help to prioritize targets for disease elimination efforts. In addition, integration of podoconiosis treatment and prevention programs with government health delivery systems is crucial to successfully eliminate the disease (Figure 6C).

9   Way Forward

As we have described in this chapter, podoconiosis is a debilitating disease common in several countries across the world. Despite its huge socio-economic and public health burden, podoconiosis has remained neglected in clinical, public health, and policy agendas until quite recently. The clinical presentation of the disease and its geographic distribution makes it distinct. The recent findings on the genetics of the disease and the experience of targeting resources to poor settings by using genetic information (family health history) are found to be effective in accelerating eradication of podoconiosis. Further investigation of the immunopathogenesis of podoconiosis will give insight into the disease mechanisms and therapeutic targets. We recommend that environmental and biomedical studies should be conducted to identify the causal environmental antigen(s) in red clay soil areas and to understand the mechanism through which these factors initiate and propagate the inflammatory immune response in genetically susceptible individuals.

Recent policy level developments shed some light into the future. For example, in 2011, the World Health Organization included podoconiosis in its list of NTDs (http://www.who.int/neglected_diseases/diseases/podoconiosis/en/). The Ethiopian Ministry of Health included podoconiosis in the National Master Plan for NTDs and in modules for the upgrading of Health Extension Workers. In addition, initiatives including Footwork - the International Podoconiosis Initiative, and the Ethiopian National Podoconiosis Action Network have been formed with vision to eliminate podoconiosis.

References

Abrahams, P. W. (2002). Soils: their implications to human health. Sci Total Environ, 291(1-3): 1-32.

Addisu, S., T. H. El-Metwally, et al. (2010). The role of transforming growth factor B1 and oxidative stress in podoconiosis pathogenesis. British J. Dermatology: DOI:10.1111/j.1365-2133.2010.09652.x.

Alemu, G., F. Tekola Ayele, et al. (2011). Burden of podoconiosis in poor rural communities in Gulliso woreda, West Ethiopia. PLoS Negl Trop Dis, 5(6): e1184.

Cohen, L. B. (1960). Idiopathic lymphoedema of Ethiopia and Kenya. East Afr Med J, 37: 53-74.

Davey, G. and E. Burridge (2009). Community-based control of a neglected tropical disease: the mossy foot treatment and prevention association. PLoS Negl Trop Dis, 3(5): e424.

Davey, G., E. Gebrehanna, et al. (2007). Podoconiosis: a tropical model for gene-environment interactions? Trans R Soc Trop Med Hyg, 101(1): 91-96.

Davey, G., F. Tekola, et al. (2007). Podoconiosis: non-infectious geochemical elephantiasis. Trans R Soc Trop Med Hyg, 101(12): 1175-1180.

Desta, K., M. Ashine, et al. (2007). Predictive value of clinical assessment of patients with podoconiosis in an endemic community setting. Trans R Soc Trop Med Hyg, 101(6): 621-623.

Destas, K., M. Ashine, et al. (2003). "Prevalence of podoconiosis (endemic non-filarial elephantiasis) in Wolaitta, Southern Ethiopia. Trop Doct, 33(4): 217-220.

Ferguson, J. S., W. Yeshanehe, et al. (2013). Assessment of skin barrier function in podoconiosis: measurement of stratum corneum hydration and transepidermal water loss. Br J Dermatol, 168(3): 550-554.

Fyfe, N. C. and E. W. Price (1985). The effects of silica on lymph nodes and vessels--a possible mechanism in the pathogenesis of non-filarial endemic elephantiasis. Trans R Soc Trop Med Hyg, 79(5): 645-651.

Geshere Oli, G., F. Tekola Ayele, et al. (2012). Parasitological, serological and clinical evidence for high prevalence of podoconiosis (non-filarial elephantiasis) in Midakegn district, central Ethiopia. Trop Med Int Health, 17(6):722-6,

Henok, L. and G. Davey (2008). Validation of the Dermatology Life Quality Index among patients with podoconiosis in southern Ethiopia. Br J Dermatol, 159(4): 903-906.

Kloos, H., A. Bedri Kello, et al. (1992). Podoconiosis (endemic non-filarial elephantiasis) in two resettlement schemes in western Ethiopia. Trop Doct, 22(3): 109-112.

Molla, Y. B., S. Tomczyk, et al. (2012a). Patients' perceptions of podoconiosis causes, prevention and consequences in East and West Gojam, Northern Ethiopia. BMC Public Health, 12: 828.

Molla, Y. B., S. Tomczyk, et al. (2012b). Podoconiosis in East and west gojam zones, northern ethiopia. PLoS Negl Trop Dis, 6(7): e1744.

Nenoff, P., J. C. Simon, et al. (2009). Podoconiosis - non-filarial geochemical elephantiasis - a neglected tropical disease? J Dtsch Dermatol Ges, 8(1): 7-14.

Oomen, A. P. (1969). A reconsideration of the problem of elephantiasis. Trop Geogr Med, 21(3): 225-235.

Oomen, A. P. (1969). Studies on elephantiasis of the legs in Ethiopia. Trop Geogr Med, 21(3): 236-253.

Price, E. (1990). Podoconiosis: Non-filarial Elephantiasis. Oxford: Oxford Medical.

Price, E. W. (1972). The pathology of non-filarial elephantiasis of the lower legs. Trans R Soc Trop Med Hyg, 66(1): 150-159.

Price, E. W. (1972). A possible genetic factor in non-filarial elephantiasis of the lower legs. Ethiop Med J, 10(3): 87-93.

Price, E. W. (1976). The association of endemic elephantiasis of the lower legs in East Africa with soil derived from volcanic rocks. Trans R Soc Trop Med Hyg, 70(4): 288-295.

Price, E. W. (1976). Endemic elephantiasis of the lower legs in Rwanda and Burundi. Trop Geogr Med, 28(4): 283-290.

Price, E. W. and W. J. Henderson (1978). The elemental content of lymphatic tissues of barefooted people in Ethiopia, with reference to endemic elephantiasis of the lower legs. Trans R Soc Trop Med Hyg, 72(2): 132-136.

Price, E. W. and W. J. Henderson (1981). Endemic elephantiasis of the lower legs in the United Cameroon Republic. Trop Geogr Med, 33(1): 23-29.

Price, E. W., W. J. McHardy, et al. (1981). Endemic elephantiasis of the lower legs as a health hazard of barefooted agriculturalists in Cameroon, West Africa. Ann Occup Hyg, 24(1): 1-8.

Sikorski, C., M. Ashine, et al. (2010). Effectiveness of a simple lymphoedema treatment regimen in podoconiosis management in southern ethiopia: one year follow-up. PLoS Negl Trop Dis, 4(11): e902.

Tekola Ayele, F., A. Adeyemo, et al. (2012). HLA class II locus and susceptibility to podoconiosis. N Engl J Med, 366(13): 1200-1208.

Tekola Ayele, F., A. Adeyemo, et al. (2012). Using a genomics tool to develop disease prevention strategy in a low-income setting: lessons from the podoconiosis research project. J Community Genet, 3(4): 303-9.

Tekola, F., S. Bull, et al. (2009). Impact of social stigma on the process of obtaining informed consent for genetic research on podoconiosis: a qualitative study. BMC Med Ethics, 10: 13.

Tekola, F., D. H. Mariam, et al. (2006). Economic costs of endemic non-filarial elephantiasis in Wolaita Zone, Ethiopia. Trop Med Int Health, 11(7): 1136-1144.

Tora, A., G. Davey, et al. (2011). A qualitative study on stigma and coping strategies of patients with podoconiosis in Wolaita zone, Southern Ethiopia. International Health, 3(3): 176-181.

Yakob, B., K. Deribe, et al. (2008). High levels of misconceptions and stigma in a community highly endemic for podoconiosis in southern Ethiopia. Trans R Soc Trop Med Hyg, 102(5): 439-444.

Yakob, B., K. Deribe, et al. (2010). Health professionals' attitudes and misconceptions regarding podoconiosis: potential impact on integration of care in southern Ethiopia. Trans R Soc Trop Med Hyg, 104(1): 42-47.

Ziegler, J. L. (1993). Endemic Kaposi's sarcoma in Africa and local volcanic soils. Lancet, 342(8883): 1348-1351.

Ziegler, J. L., T. Simonart, et al. (2001). Kaposi's sarcoma, oncogenic viruses, and iron. J Clin Virol, 20(3): 127-130.

Evaluation of Morning and Evening Nasal Symptoms Scores of Allergic Rhinitis: A Pooled-Analysis of Rupatadine Randomized Placebo-Controlled Clinical Trials

Iñaki Izquierdo
Clinical Development & Medical Advisory Department
J Uriach y Compañia S.A, Barcelona, Catalonia, Spain

Josep Giralt
Clinical Development & Medical Advisory Department
J Uriach y Compañia S.A, Barcelona, Catalonia, Spain

Alejandro Doménech
Clinical Development & Medical Advisory Department
J Uriach y Compañia S.A, Barcelona, Catalonia, Spain

1   Introduction

Many inflammatory diseases exhibit variations in symptoms over time. Specifically, symptoms of allergic rhinitis (AR) have been shown to follow a pattern of circadian variation (Storms, 2004). Thus, severity of symptoms of AR is typically greater in the morning for all major symptoms, including nasal blockage, runny nose and sneezing, in approximately 70% of patients (Haye *et al.*, 2005). Possible causes of increased morning symptoms include increased levels of histamine and other inflammatory mediators (Aoyagi *et al.*, 1999). Patients report that morning symptoms have a negative impact on quality of life throughout the rest of the day. Therefore, an important consideration in the pharmacologic treatment of AR is the effective relief of morning symptoms.

Second-generation oral antihistamines are among the most widely prescribed agents due to their effectiveness in the treatment of allergic diseases. Although newer long-acting antihistamine preparations permit once-daily dosing, many patients with AR experience breakthrough symptoms and a reduction of clinical efficacy at the end of the dosing interval. Most antihistamines demonstrate a peak effect approximately 5 to 7 hours after oral administration, and the duration varies depending on the half-life of parent compound and active metabolites (Brunton, 2002).

The aim of this study was to evaluate the overall efficacy of rupatadine, an anti-H_1 and PAF antagonist compound (Keam & Plosker, 2007; Merlos *et al.*, 1997; Mullol *et al.*, 2008), in the control of morning and evening nasal symptoms in patients with allergic rhinitis.

2   Methods

This analysis includes the pooled data from five randomized, double blind, placebo-controlled studies previously published as separate trials (Fantin *et al.*, 2008; Guadaño *et al.*, 2004; Izquierdo *et al.*, 2000; Lukat *et al.*, 2013; Marmouz *et al.*, 2011). These studies had approximately the same number of patients as well as a similar study design, which makes the pooled analysis appropriate. The only difference among the studies was the treatment duration, which was longer (12 weeks) for one study in Perennial AR (PAR) compared to the 2 and 4-week duration for the rest of the trials All patients received 10 mg od (1 tablet rupatadine) or placebo od, both tablets had the same appearance and were packaged identically.

2.1   Inclusion and Exclusion Criteria

Inclusion and exclusion criteria were very similar between trials. Patients aged $\geq$ 18 years old with a diagnosis of AR for at least 12 months, and with a total nasal symptom score $\geq$ 5 (out of a possible total score of 12) were included in the study. During a screening visit, the patients must show a positive skin prick test (diameter of the papule > 3 mm compared to saline solution control, or $\geq$ to that obtained with histamine at a 10 mg/mL dilution) at inclusion or within one year before inclusion. The allergens used in the prick test are usually related to PAR or SAR. A normal 12-lead ECG had to be documented at the pre-screening visit with the following requirements: QTc < 430 msec for males, and QTc < 450 msec for females. Women of childbearing age had to show a negative pregnancy test and had to use contraceptive measures during the study.

Patients suffering from non-allergic rhinitis (e.g. vasomotor, infectious or drug-induced rhinitis) or with a negative prick test were not included. Treatments with nasal descongestionants in the previous 24 hours, oral antihistamines or disodium chromoglycate (previous week), ketotifen (previous month), topical antihistamines (previous 48 hours), systemic or topical treatment with corticosteroids (except for topical hydrocortisone < 1%), immunosuppressants, or any investigational drug taken within 2 weeks prior to inclusion were considered as exclusion criteria. Other relevant exclusion criteria included abnormal laboratory values (including hematology and blood chemistry tests) of clinical significance, certain conditions that may interfere with response to treatment such as mild asthma treated with inhaled bronchodilators or inhaled corticosteroids (> 800 mcg/day of budesonide or beclomethasone, or > 500 mcg/day of fluticasone), obstructive nasal polyps or hypersensitivity to compounds structurally related to the study drug.

2.2   Evaluation of Efficacy

In order to compare across studies, the primary endpoint variable was defined as the mean change from baseline of total reflective symptoms' score (T4SS) at 2, 4, 8 and 12 weeks of treatment duration. We used the total nasal symptoms' score since this has been suggested to be a much more appropriate measure for allergic rhinitis symptoms assessment (European Medicines Agency, 2005). T4SS consists of a composite score of the severity scores for four AR symptoms (runny nose, itchy nose, blocked nose and sneezing), which were recorded in patient dairy cards. Each symptom was scored 0-3 (with 0=absent, 1=mild, 2=moderate, or 3=severe) twice daily, in the morning (AM) within 1 h of awakening and prior to drug intake and in the evening (PM), around 12 h later. Both the AM and PM symptom severity were assessed in a reflective manner (over the previous 12 h).

Additional the safety of treatments were evaluated accordingly to the incidence of adverse events (AEs) recorded in the patient's diaries. All AEs were coded using the same MedDRA dictionary across all clinical studies.

Daily AM/PM symptoms scores were analyzed from a fixed effect model, weighting the average of each study scores by its individual variance and the subject evaluation was carried out with Cochran's Mantel-Haenszel test. All statistical procedures were performed using SAS® software version 9.1 for Windows (SAS Institute Inc. Cary, NC USA). All tests of significance were carried out at a 0.05 level.

3   Results

Table 1 summarizes the main features of the five controlled clinical trials included in this pooled analysis. A total of 1017 patients (RUP=511; PBO=506) were included in the pooled analysis at baseline score.

Rupatadine showed a significant reduction of symptoms' score at AM and PM evaluations. The mean change from baseline over 2, 4, 8 and 12 weeks of the TSS morning (AM) evaluations showed significant improvements ($p < 0.001$) in the ANOVA comparison with placebo group (see Figure 1). Reductions from baseline of -35%, -40%, -49% and -55% were obtained at 2,4,8, and 12 weeks respectively. Similarly, the mean change from baseline of the TSS evening (PM) evaluations were also significant ($p < 0.001$) at 2 (-32%), 8 (-41%) and 12 (-49%) weeks, with the exception of 4 (-41%) weeks, which was not significant (see Figure 2).

When individual symptoms were assessed, statistically significant improvement for runny nose was detected in the morning (AM) evaluation at 2 ($p < 0.001$), 4 ($p < 0.05$), 8 ($p < 0.001$) and 12 ($p < 0.001$) weeks (see figure 3a). The evening (PM) evaluations showed only significant improvement for this symptom at 2 ($p < 0.001$) and 12 ($p < 0.001$) weeks (see figure 3b). The itchy nose showed statistically significant improvements at any time: 2 ($p < 0.001$), 4 ($p < 0.05$), 8 ($p < 0.001$) and 12 weeks ($p <$

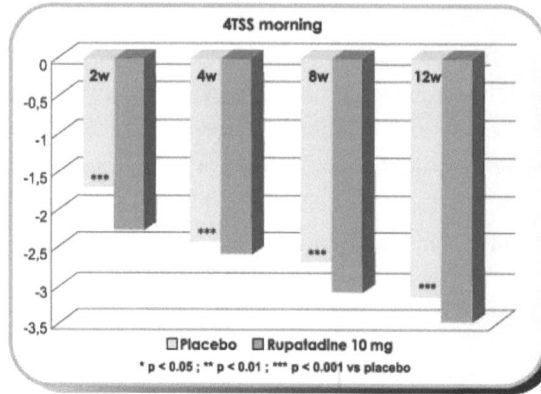

Figure 1: 4TSS morning (AM evaluation). Mean change from baseline over 2, 4, 8 and 12 weeks.

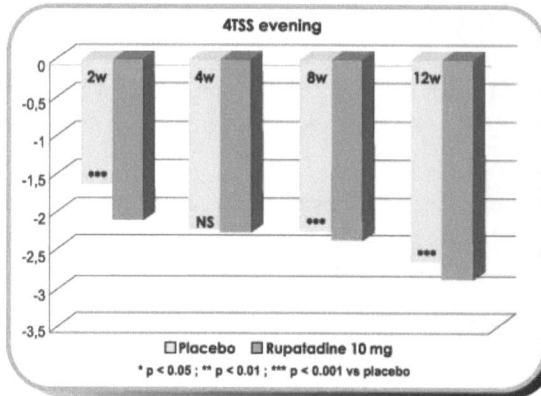

Figure 2: 4TSS evening (PM evaluation). Mean change from baseline over 2, 4, 8 and 12 weeks.

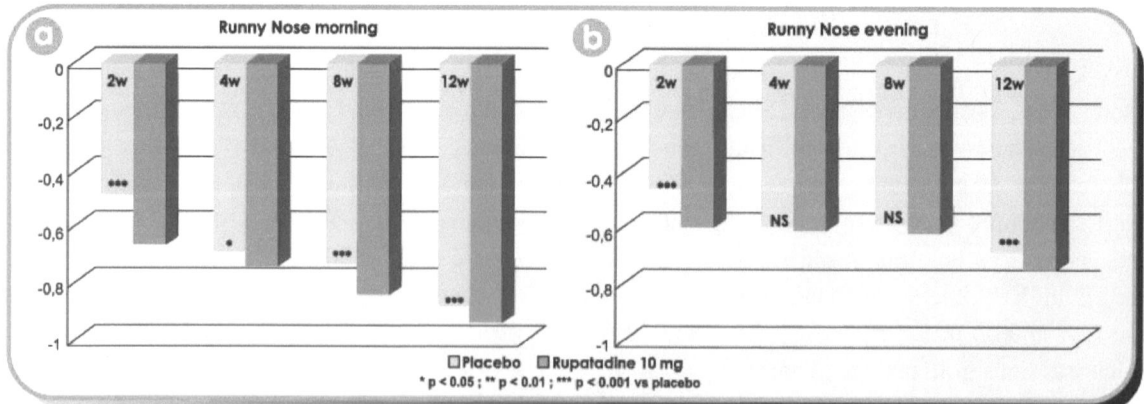

Figure 3: Runny nose. (a) Morning: AM evaluation; **(b)** Evening: PM evaluation. Mean change from baseline over 2, 4, 8 and 12 weeks.

Treatment groups	Allergic Rhinitis	N Patients	Duration (weeks)	Study Design / Level of Evidence	Age (Years) Mean ± sd	Reference
Rupatadine 10 mg od Rupatadine 20 mg od Placebo od	SAR	178	2	m, r, db, pg, Level 2	35 ± 12.7	Izquierdo *et al.*, 2000
Rupatadine 10 mg od Ebastine10 mg od Placebo od	SAR	250	2	m, r, db, pg, Level 2	33 ± 10.1	Guadaño *et al.*, 2004
Rupatadine 10 mg od Desloratadine 5 mg od Placebo od	SAR	379	4	m, r, db, pg, Level 2	31 ± 12.7	Lukat *et al.*, 2013
Rupatadine 10 mgl od Rupatadine 20 mg od Cetirizine10 mg od Placebo od	PAR	282	4	m, r, db, pg, Level 2	32 ± 10.9	Marmouz *et al.*, 2011
Rupatadine 10 mg od Cetirizine 10 mg od Placebol od	PER	543	12	m, r, db, pg Level 2	29 ± 12.9	Fantin *et al.*, 2008

Table 1: SAR; seasonal allergic rhinitis; PAR, perennial allergic rhinitis; PER persistent allergic rhinitis ; m, multicentre; r, randomized, db, double-blind, pg, parallel groups, od, once daily.

0.001) (see figure 4a). On the contrary when the PM evaluation was analyzed, the improvement was significant only the first 2 weeks ($p < 0.001$) (see figure 4b). Nasal obstruction was also evaluated at morning achieving clear significant improvements at 2 ($p < 0.001$), 4 ($p < 0.001$), 8 ($p < 0.001$) and 12 weeks ($p < 0.001$) (see figure 5a). The evening evaluations for blocked nose showed an important and consistent improvement at 2 ($p < 0.001$), 4 ($p < 0.001$), 8 ($p < 0.001$) and 12 weeks ($p < 0.01$) as well (see figure 5b). The last symptom evaluated was sneezing, which is one of the most common symptoms in AR. The morning evaluations showed significant improvements at 2 ($p < 0.001$), 4 ($p < 0.001$), 8 ($p < 0.001$) and 12 weeks ($p < 0.001$) (see figure 6a), while in the evening evaluations a significant improvement were detected at 2 ($p < 0.001$), 4 ($p < 0.001$) and 12 weeks ($p < 0.001$) (see figure 6b).

Finally, the change in score from baseline after the first 12 h was also evaluated, showing runny nose, itchy nose and sneezing as significantly ($p < 0.001$) better than placebo.

The total AEs incidences was 25%(n=126) for patients taking placebo and 38% (n=194) and for rupatadine 10 mg ($p < 0.01$). Both groups of treatment showed a similar pattern of safety, including some side effects in gastrointestinal and SNC systems. Only the incidence of somnolence was statistically significant with rupatadine in comparison with placebo ($p < 0.01$).

4   Discussion

The second generation of anti-H_1 antihistamines play an important role in the treatment of AR at all severity stages, and are indeed recommended by current guidelines (Bousquet *et al.*, 2008).

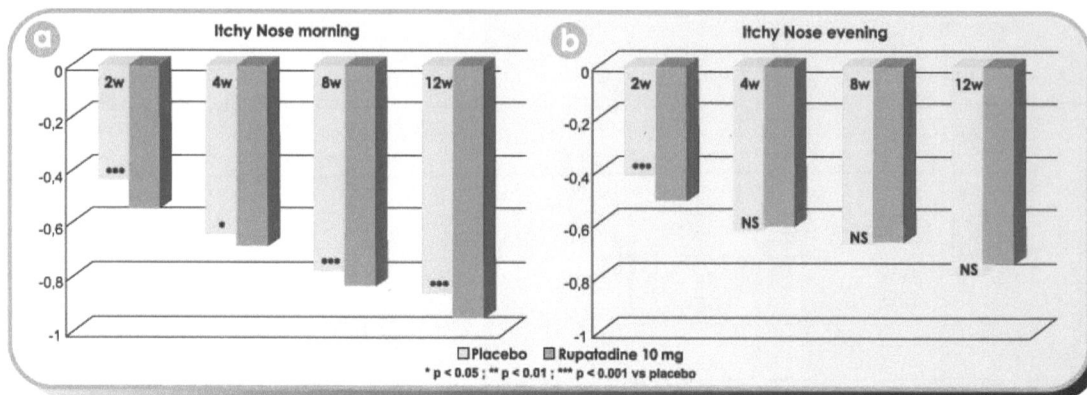

Figure 4: Itching nose. (a) Morning: AM evaluation; (b) Evening: PM evaluation. Mean change from baseline over 2, 4, 8 and 12 weeks.

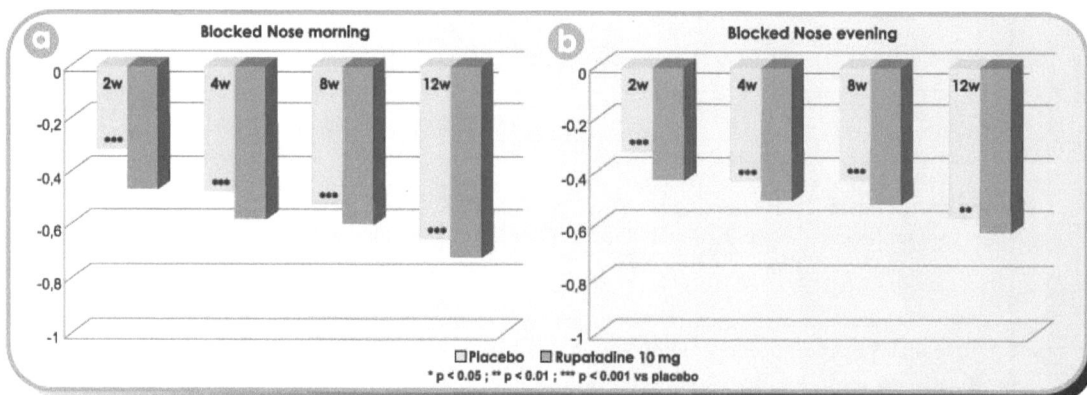

Figure 4: Blocked nose. (a) Morning: AM evaluation; (b) Evening: PM evaluation. Mean change from baseline over 2, 4, 8 and 12 weeks.

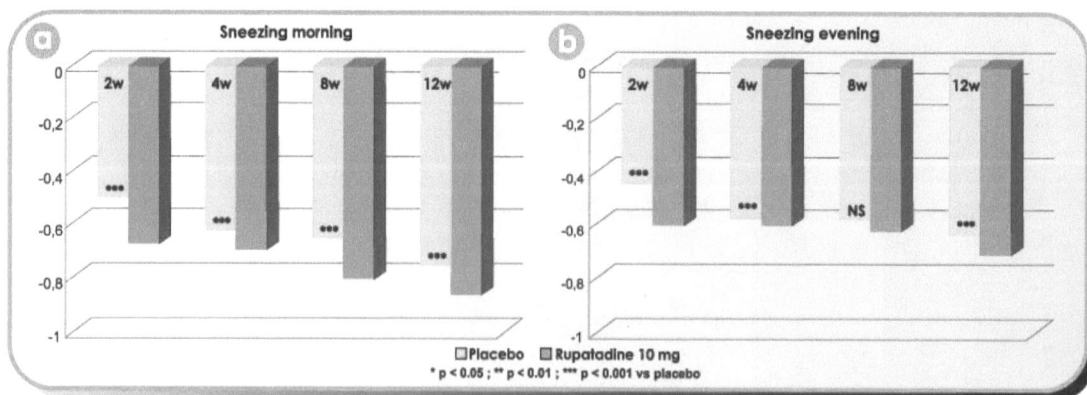

Figure 6: Sneezing. (a) Morning: AM evaluation; (b) Evening: PM evaluation. Mean change from baseline over 2, 4, 8 and 12 weeks.

The symptoms of AR vary in severity over the course of the day and are often worse in the morning. Actually, the intensity of nasal congestion, rhinorrhea and sneezing are greater early in the morning in approximately 70 % of patients (Schenkel, 2006; Smolensky et al., 1995). This is true for patients with seasonal symptoms alone (55.9%) and also for those with PAR (65.7%), although it is noteworthy that those with PAR reported worse symptoms in the morning significantly more often than those with SAR (Binder et al., 1982). Therefore, in order to maximize the benefits for patients and also to maintain a good overall efficacy profile, any pharmacologic agent used in the management of allergic rhinitis should be effective in controlling these peak morning symptoms. In general, antihistamines would be expected to exert their maximum effect near or shortly after peak serum levels are reached. In the case of rupatadine, previous studies showed a fast on-set of action (Mullol et al. 2008), due to the fact that levels reach its peak serum levels around 0.5 – 1 hour after dosing (Keam et al., 2007). This was the main reason why morning dosageas scheduled in our study and so we expected to observe a greater relief of morning symptoms in comparison with those evening symptoms. Notably, in our study, the overall (T4SS) relief of symptoms was quite similar for AM or PM period with rupatadine 10 mg once daily, indicating a sustained 24-hour effect of rupatadine irrespective of time of dosing. These 4TSS values are in concordance with previous clinical controlled studies of rupatadine using active controls (Fantin et al., 2008; Lukat et al., 2013).

When individual nasal symptoms were evaluated at AM or PM, different patterns were observed. The morning evaluations showed all symptoms' scores well controlled, with a high significant improvement in all treatment periods (from 2 to 12 weeks). Specifically, a significant capacity to alleviate sneezing and nasal blockage in the morning was provided by rupatadine in all evaluated periods. Nasal congestion is a particularly troublesome symptom of allergic rhinitis and is often cited by patients as the most bothersome one. Newer antihistamines have demonstrated anti-inflammatory properties which could play a role in the control of nasal inflammation. However the results of their effects clinical trials on nasal congestion are not enough conclusive (Horak, 2002). Rupatadine was previously shown to reduce nasal congestion effectively in patients with SAR, having been measured, both objectively in terms of nasal airflow or subjectively in terms of symptoms in allergen exposure study (Stübner et al., 2006; Valero et al., 2009).

The nighttime symptoms are an important component of the total morbiditty associated with AR[1]. Both sleep disorders and AR are associated with increases in daytime somnolence, fatigue, irritability, absenteeism and performance impairment. It is clear that nasal itching and runny nose do not improve sleep quality; however, nasal congestion is thought to be the main symptom responsible for rhinitis-related sleep problems (Juniper et al., 2003).

In our analysis of the nigttimesymptoms, runny nose and itchy nose were not well controlled, and actually they did not achieve statistically significant improvements in comparison with placebo. These findings may be explained in part by the fact that these symptoms were most likely underreported (by the patients) in the clinical trials. Additionally, it seems that there was not enough statistical power to found significant differences between both group's scores. Sneezing and nasal blockage are symptoms which may be particularly troublesome for patients at nighttime. Sneezing could delay the onset of sleep and nasal blockage, subsequent to nasal congestion, can lead to pathologic changes in airflow velocity and increase the sleep-disordered breathing (Young et al., 1998). In our pooled analysis rupatadine reduce the szeening and nasal blockage at nighttime e in comparison with placebo.

In relation with the incidence of side effects, was low and most of them have been previously reported with antiH1 second generation, like gastrointestinal and central nervous system side effects. Mild somnolence episodes were more frequent related with rupatadine treatment. There was a consistent low frequency of somnolence across the studies in those patients receiving rupatadine (Fantin *et al.*, 2011; Guadaño *et al.*, 2004; Izquierdo *et al.*, 2000; Lukat *et al.*, 2013; Marmouz *et al.*, 2011).

The specific underlying mechanisms of the chronobiology of AR are not clear established; however, several factors might contribute to the occurrence of maximum nasal blockage, sneezing and rhinorrhea in the morning: secretions increase and accumulate overnight; there is continuous allergen exposure to mold, mites or house dander; cortisol levels are lowest at night, and hence inflammatory mediators might be at high levels; and autonomic nervous system activity at night promotes vagal tone, favoring vasodilation (Meltzer, 2002).

In this analysis, rupatadine maintains its effect throughout the day and at different periods of treatment duration (from 2 to 12 weeks) and apparently shows no circadian variation of effect when the symptoms are globally evaluated. This activity could be explained by an additional and sustained anti-inflammatory effect of rupatadine (Mullol *et al.*, 2008). These patients have a continuous inflammation in the nose caused by the persistent allergen exposure throughout the years. This concept of a minimal persistent inflammation would involve, at least in theory, several mediators produced by primary effector cells, which would play an important role in the onset and maintenance of the inflammatory allergic process (Ciprandi *et al.*, 1995). As a consequence, active drugs like rupatadine, capable of interfering with more than one class of these mediators, could provide a better control for allergic inflammatory symptoms in comparison with other anti-H_1 compounds which have not this simultaneous blocking capacity (Fantin *et al.*, 2008).

In conclusion, the sustained 24-hour action of rupatadine 10 mg provides an effective control of morning and evening symptoms from 2 up to 12-weeks of treatment in patients with several subtypes of allergic rhinitis.

Competing interests

The study was funded by J Uriach y Compañia, S.A (Barcelona, Spain). The authors are employees of Clinical development Dept at J Uriach Company.

Author's contributions

II participated in the design of study, analysis interpretation and drafting of the manuscript.
JG participated in the statistical analysis, the tables and figures preparation and drafting the manuscript.
AD participated in the analysis interpretation and reviewing the manuscript.

References

Storms W W. (2004). *Pharmacologic approaches to daytime and nighttime symptoms of allergic rhinitis. J Allergy Clin Immunol. 2004; 114 (Suppl):S146-S153.*

Haye R, Høye K, Berg O, et al. (2005). *Morning versus evening dosing of desloratadine in seasonal allergic rhinitis: a randomized controlled study. Clin Mol Allergy. 2005; 3:1-6.*

Aoyagi M, Watanabe H, Sekine K, et al. (1999). Circadian variation in nasal reactivity in children with allergic rhinitis: correlation with the activity of eosinophils and basophilic cells. Int Arch Allergy Immunol. 1999;120 Suppl 1:95-9.

Brunton SA. (2002). Allergy management strategies: An update. Patient Care. 2002; spring (suppl):16-25.

Merlos M, Giral M, Balsa D, et al. (1997). Rupatadine, a new potent, orally active dual antagonist of histamine and platelet-activating factor (PAF). J Pharmacol Exp Ther. 1997;280(1):114-121.

Mullol J, Bousquet J, Bachert C, et al. (2008). Rupatadine in allergic rhinitis and chronic urticaria. Allergy 2008: 63 (Suppl. 87):5-28.

Keam SJ, Plosker GL. (2007). Rupatadine: a review of its use in the management of allergic disorders. Drug. 2007; 67(3):457-74.

Izquierdo I, Paredes I, Lurigados C, Sospedra E; Cooper M, Thomas H. (2000). A dose ranging study of rupatadine fumarate in patients with seasonal allergic rhinitis. Allergy 2000; 55 (Suppl 63): 275.

Guadaño EM, Serra Batlles J, Meseguer J, Castillo JA, de Molina M, Valero A, Picado C. (2004). Rupatadine 10 mg and ebastine 10 mg in seasonal allergic rhinitis: a comparison study. Allergy 2004; 59 (7): 766-71.

Marmouz F, Giralt J, Izquierdo I. (2011). Rupatadine investigator's group. Morning and evening efficacy evaluation of rupatadine (10 and 20 mg), compared with cetirizine 10 mg in perennial allergic rhinitis: a randomized, double-blind, placebo-controlled trial. J Asthma Allergy 2011; 4 :27–35.

Fantin S, Maspero J, Bisbal C, Agache I, Donado E, Borja J, Mola O, Izquierdo I. (2008). A 12-week placebo-controlled study of rupatadine 10 mg once daily compared with cetirizine 10 mg once daily, in the treatment of persistent allergic rhinitis. Allergy 2008; 63 (7): 924-931.

Lukat KF, Rivas P, Roger A, Kowalski ML, Botzen U, Wessel F, Sanquer F, Agache I, Izquierdo I. (2013). A direct comparison of efficacy between desloratadine and rupatadine in seasonal allergic rhinoconjunctivitis: a randomized, double-blind, placebo-controlled study. J Asthma Allergy 2013; 6: 31-9.

European Medicines Agency. (2005). Guideline on the clinical development of medicinal products for the treatment of allergic rhino-conjunctivitis. London, UK; Committee for medicinal products for human use; 2005. Available from: http://www.ema.europa.eu/docs/en_GB/document_library/Scientific_guideline/2009/09/WC500003554.pdf.

Bousquet J, Khaltaev N, Cruz AA, et al. (2008). Allergic Rhinitis and its Impact on Asthma (ARIA) 2008 update (in collaboration with the World Health Organization, GA(2)LEN and AllerGen). Allergy. 2008; 63 Suppl 86:8-160.

Smolensky NH, Reinberg A, Labrecque G. (1995). Twenty-four hour pattern in symptom intensity of viral and allergic rhinitis: treatment implications. J Allergy Clin Inmunol. 1995; 95:1084-96.

Schenkel E. (2006). Effect of desloratadine on the control of morning symtomps in patients with seasonal and perennial allergic rhinitis. Allergy Asthma. 2006; Proc 27:465-472.

Binder E, Holopainen E, Malmberg H, Salo O. (1982). Anamnestic data in allergic rhinitis. Allergy. 1982; 37:389-396.

Horak F. Impact and modulation of nasal obstruction. Allergy 2002; 57 Suppl 75:25-28.

Valero A, Serrano C, Bartrá J, et al. (2009). Reduction of nasal volume after allergen-induced rhinitis in patients treated with rupatadine: a randomized, cross-over, double-blind, placebo-controlled study. Investig Allergol Clin Immunol. 2009;19(6):488-93.

Stübner P, Horak F, Zieglmayer R, et al. (2006). Effects of rupatadine vs placebo on allergen-induced symptoms in patients exposed to aeroallergens in the Vienna Challenge Chamber. Ann Allergy Asthma Immunol. 2006;96(1):37-44.

Juniper EF, Rohrbaugh T, Meltzer EO. (2003). A questionnaire to measure quality of life in adults with nocturnal allergic rhinoconjunctivitis. J Allergy Clin Inmunol 2003; 111(suppl): S835-42.

Young T, Finn L, Kim H. (1998). University of Wisconsin Sleep nas respiratory Research Group. nsal obstruction as a risk factor for sleep-disordered breathing. J Allergy Clin Inmunol 1998; 101:633-7.

Meltzer EO. (2002). Does rhinitis compromise nigh-time sleep and daytime productivity ? Clin Exp Allergy Rev. 2002; 2:67-72.

Ciprandi G, Buscaglia S, Pesce G, Pronzato C, Ricca V, Parmiani S et al. (1995). Minimal persistent inflammation is present at mucosal level in patients with asymptomatic rhinitis and mite allergy. J Allergy Clin Inmunol 1995; 96: 971-979.

Occupational and Environmental Risk Factors for Allergic and Hypersensitivity Reactions

Hülya Gül

Department of Public Health, Istanbul Medical Faculty
Istanbul University, Istanbul, Turkey

Zahide Ceren Atli

University of California, Berkeley, USA

1   Introduction

Nowadays, allergic disease is accepted as a significant public health problem which is frequently observed worldwide. In recent times, the mechanism of allergic disease has focused on the genetic and environment interaction. So, it is important to consider the occupational and environmental risk factors of allergic disease. Allergy is no longer considered to be solely related with heritage, but the negative effects of modern life due to technological developments are accepted as important factors in the etiology. An allergy is a hypersensitivity reaction of a person to the environment, described as the surroundings to which it is exposed. Allergic reactions are not of one type, they can be created in various ways, can develop in various body regions and differ in severity. These allergic substances can be exposed to the airway, skin contact or taken orally with foods.

Environmental allergic risk factors can affect people at any age from childhood. Health complaints related to allergy are commonly seen in the general population. It has been reported that allergic conditions are present in 10% of the community in the USA, in 15-30% in European countries, and in 9-20% in Turkey according to different studies (Pawankar et al., 2011; Greiner 2011; Kurt et al., 2009). However, these rates have increased over time, especially in industrialized countries. Allergy affects the quality of life of people in a markedly negative way by disrupting their health. For example, in recent decades, allergic eye problems have frequently been a major health problem for workers. One of the main symptoms of allergy is ocular symptoms: irritation, foreign body sensation and dryness. The work climate has changed a lot and employees are very dependent on their eyes in the office during the working day. Many workers have allergic eye symptoms in chemical metal factories and paint shops. There are some people who only have work related allergy symptoms in their eyes (e.g., latex powder from gloves, tree dust in joineries etc.). Also, air conditioning plays a more important role in many work places than previously thought. Air conditioning is one of the main sources for many kinds of allergic or allergy-like eye problems, allergic conjunctivitis and dry eye. Problems with the internal air of buildings directly affect eyes that are the most sensitive part of the body. At the same time, allergy is notably one of the main reasons for school and work absenteeism.

Allergic reactions are not of a single type, they occur by many ways, may involve different parts of the body, and may be of varying severity. Although the term allergy suggests symptoms including pruritus in the skin, nasal discharge and sneezing, many different allergic conditions occur depending on the organ involved and the agent affecting the individual. These conditions mainly include allergic rhinitis, allergic bronchial asthma, allergic coryza and conjunctivitis, cutaneous allergy, food allergy, drug allergy, insect allergy, and occupational allergies arising from substances found in the workplace. Allergic rhinitis is a high prevalence morbidity affecting 10-20% of the general population in many developed countries (Asher et al., 2006). Allergic rhinitis is divided into three subgroups; continuous, seasonal and occupational, depending on the time or place of exposure to allergens. Perennial allergic rhinitis occurs most commonly with house dust mites and animal dander. Seasonal allergic rhinitis occurs due to hay fields or different tree pollens. The morbidity of seasonal allergic rhinitis depends on the geographical region, the pollen season of plants, and local climatic conditions.

Allergic diseases occur commonly in childhood (Jackson et al., 2013). Approximately one out of every four children in the world has an allergic disease (asthma, allergic rhinitis, allergic eczema, food allergy, drug allergy, insect allergy, or urticaria). The allergic influences of environmental conditions in humans start before birth, during pregnancy of the mother. Most commonly, exposure during childhood has a negative influence on the developmental prognosis and life too. The factors involved in the occurrence of an allergy in children's future include the mother's nutrition, whether the mother smokes, and the level of pollution in the environment during the intrauterine period. Many studies have proven that environmental factors including smoking and passive smoking during pregnancy increase the risk of both asthma and allergy in children (Dotterud *et al.*, 2013). In addition, the presence of intensive humidity in the household may later trigger the development of asthma. Also, among the important factors that determine whether a child will be allergic or not are nutrition after birth, the presence of breastfeeding and even the mode of delivery (normal vaginal or cesarean). Children, especially those with asthma, get tired more quickly, sweat and cough more compared with their peers from the early periods of life. Some causal triggers for this disease include surroundings that contain allergens or air pollution, influenza, work environment, chemical residues on clothing, intense odors, and excessive exercise (Friis *et al.*, 2013).

Currently, allergies are not addressed only in relation with the genetic predisposition, but the role of the negative impact of modern life conditions is being discussed more intensely. Many factors which cause allergy are not harmful at a level that threatens life, and they do not necessarily lead to discomfort or have an impact in one hundred percent of people. Studies show that genetics and environmental factors are involved together in the occurrence of the disease (Carlsten & Melen 2012; Kauffmann *et al.*, 2012; Mutius, 2004). A gene-environment interaction occurs in this disease at a high rate. Thus, allergic diseases can be defined as an eco-genetic phenomenon with in this regard. Allergic diseases are characterized with an abnormal immune response to environmental antigens which are confronted frequently. Substances which trigger allergic reactions and lead to allergic reactions are called allergic substances or allergens. These substances can be taken in by the respiratory tract, by skin contact or by the oral route with foods. Allergy symptoms may be transient for some people and continuous for others. These range from transient discomfort to severe and life-threatening conditions, including severe asthma. Symptoms change from person to person. Inadequate diagnosis and treatment can lead to more frequent attacks.

This section of the book discusses environmental and occupational risk factors which are thought to a great extent to be responsible for allergic diseases, with an emphasis on the role of indoor and outdoor air pollution, preservatives in our foods and unfavorable workplace conditions. Based on the epidemiological data in developed and developing countries, we aim to draw attention to the current status and new ways of understanding allergies and propose solutions for the future.

2 Prevalence

In recent years, there has been an increase in the prevalence of allergic diseases, especially in developed countries (Wong *et al.*, 2013; Hong S., 2012). Allergic diseases are observed more commonly in industrialized countries compared with agricultural countries, and in urban populations compared with rural populations (Ghosh *et al.*, 2013). Environmental pollution, climate change, preservatives in foods, new generation drugs, and rapid industrial developments have all been shown to cause this increase (Barnes *et al*, 2013; Thong & Tan, 2011). The unfavorable factors which are continuously present in an individual's life including pollutants in drinking water, foods, and indoor and outdoor air, inhibit or weaken the immune system and render an individual more sensitive to allergenic substances. The World Allergy Organization reported that 22% of the participants in global scale studies (approximately 250 million people) suffered from at least one of the allergic diseases. These studies were conducted with approximately 1.39 billion individuals in 33 countries (Warner *et al.*, 2006). In Turkey, allergic asthma has been found with a rate of

2- to 5%, allergic rhinitis and allergic eczema have been found with a rate of 0.08% and food allergies have been found with a rate of 5% (Dinmezel, 2005; Emri, 2005). Asthma has also shown a significant increase in Turkey (TUİK, 2013; T.C. 2009; Ones, 2006). In addition, according to recent evidence, it has been emphasized that only 1/3 of asthma cases use to occur as a result of allergic causes 30 years ago, but this rate has currently reached 80% (Kauppi *et al.*, 2013; Wertz, 2010). The World Health Organization reports that there are about 300 million asthma patients worldwide. Each year, 180,000 individuals lose their lives because of this disease worldwide. In the USA, it has been reported that the number of asthma patients has shown a significant increase of 60% since 1980 (Akinbami *et al.*, 2012; Moorman *et al.*, 2012).

3   Occupational and Environmental Risk Factors

Risk factors for an allergy can be evaluated in two categories including host factors and environmental factors. As with many diseases, allergic diseases also occur when adequate environmental factors are present on an appropriate genetic background (Wang, 2005; Okatria *et al.*, 2013; Pleil *et al.*, 2012; Shah, 2012). Many individual factors including heredity, sex, race and age may regulate an allergy. There are many different allergens. Among these, the most common ones and the ones which lead to allergic disease include environmental allergens (D'amato *et al.*, 2010; Kurt, 2010). Environmental factors include foods, clothes, air, water, detergents, cleaning materials, chemicals in the workplace (Kim *et al.*, 2013; Moual *et al*, 2008; Peden, 2010). These are divided as indoor and outdoor factors by their localization. The reason that this differentiation is made is that the type and findings of allergic disease varies according to the type of allergen. For example, the most common indoor allergen is house mites which are found in house dust. Mites lead to allergies throughout the whole year, in all four seasons. In contrast, outdoor allergens include mainly hay fields, tree and flower pollens which mostly lead to allergies in the spring. Individuals may also be exposed to other allergens including foods, drugs and insects, which do not precisely fit in this classification due to differing time periods and settings. Allergic contact urticaria and contact dermatitis/eczema, occupational asthma and rhinitis are one of the most common occupational allergic skin and respiratory diseases. Occupational allergies are new emerging diseases that seen among workers who exposed to allergic substances in the workplace environment. Occupational allergic diseases are common with a prevalence of % 5 -15 in the worldwide. As can be seen in Table 1, 2, 3, 4 chemicals, physical agents etc., a lot of substances used at work can cause the allergy (Vandenplas *et al.*, 2011; Peden & Reed 2010; Wick, 2013).

The occurrence of allergic diseases has increased in parallel with the changes in modern life style in urban regions. It was thought that industrial sources and environmental pollution were responsible for this. In diseases which occur as a result of unfavorable environmental factors, therapy can be provided not only by way of drugs, but also by way of investigations to find the environmental causes of the disease, eradication of these causes and increasing the resistance of the patient (Yeşillik & Öztürk, 2013). The most important point in the protection from allergies is the determination and eradication of suspicious environmental allergens in closed settings such as houses and workplaces where the individual lives, or reducing contact with these allergens to a minimum.

Occupation	Allergens
Contact dermatitis:	
Bakers	Flavoring, oil, antioxidant
Building trade workers	Cement (Cr, Co), rubber, resin, wood
Caterers, cooks	Vegetable/fruit, cutlery (Ni), rubber gloves, spice
Cleaners	Rubber gloves, nickel, fragrance
Dental personnel	Rubber, acrylate, fragrance, mercury
Electronics assemblers	Cr, Co, Ni, acrylate, epoxy resin
Hairdressers	Dye, rubber, fragrance, Ni, thioglycolate
Metal workers	Preservative, Ni, Cr, Co, antioxidant
Office workers	Rubber, Ni, dye, glue, copying paper
Textile workers	Formaldehyde resin, dye, Ni
Veterinarians, farmers	Rubber, antibiotics, plants, preservatives
Contact urticaria:	
Cooks	Animal products, wheat, vegetables
Health-care providers	Latex
Hair dressers	Dyes, latex
Animal workers	Animal dander

Table 1: Allergens and occupations causing contact dermatitis and urticaria

Agent	Occupation/industry
Cereals, flour	Flour mills, bakers, pastry makers, the Mediterranean flour moth
Latex	Health-care workers, laboratory technicians
Enzymes	Baking products production, bakers, detergent production, pharmaceutical industry, food industry
Animals	Laboratory workers, farmers, sea foods processing
Isocyanates	Polyurethane production, plastic industry, moulding, spray painters
Metals	Metal refinery, metal alloy production, electroplating, welding
Biocides	Health-care workers, cleaners
Reactive dyes	Textile workers, food industry workers
Woods	Sawmill workers, carpenters, cabinet and furniture

Table 2: Principal Agents Causing Occupational Asthma, Rhinitis and Conjunctivitis

High molecular weight	Low molecular weight
Grain dust (including mites)	Diisocyanates (many sources)
Bakery dust	Acid anhydrides
Fish proteins	Western red cedar (plicatic acid)
Laboratory animals	Colophony
Bird proteins	Penicillin
Natural rubber latex	Nickel
Enzymes, especially detergents	Platinum
Mold proteins	Vanadium
Vegetable gums	
Soy bean dust	
Cotton, coffee, and other seed dusts	
Psyllium	

Table 3: Some common occupational allergens due to molecular weight

Occupation	Potential Allergen and Manifestation
Bakery and Food Service Workers	Wheat flour exposure can cause respiratory (*e.g.*, rhinitis, nasal allergies, etc.) and eye symptoms or a systemic reaction Soy beans, fish, shellfish, and egg can cause systemic reaction Peanut-based products can cause systemic allergic reaction
Carpenters and Wood Workers	Exotic hardwoods can cause rhinitis, asthma, or contact dermatitis
Chemical and Pharmaceutical Factory Workers	Enzymes, medication, and biological dusts can cause sensitivity allergy Ammonia, bleach, and chloramines can cause rhinitis
Cleaning Staff	Bleaches and enzymes from detergents can cause contact dermatitis or asthma
Electrical Workers	Fumes from soldering may cause lung disease
Engine Mechanics	Benzene can cause contact dermatitis
Farm Workers, Dockworkers, and Cotton Workers	Moldy hay stored in silos can cause hypersensitivity pnuemonitis (now rare) Poultry and plant dusts can cause asthma
Florists	Primula, ivy, and lilies can cause contact dermatitis
Hairdressers	Paraphenylene diamine in dyes and bleaches can cause contact dermatitis and eczema Persulfates in permanent wave solution can cause respiratory distress or dermatitis or eczema
Laboratory Workers	Animal dander, saliva components, or bird proteins can cause asthma Endotoxins can cause asthma Solvent vapors and inorganic acid vapors or mist may cause rhinitis
Laborers	Chromium in cement can cause contact dermatitis
Medical Workers	Latex rubber in gloves, tubing, and medical supplies can cause contact dermatitis
Miners	Coal dust can cause nasal symptoms or chronic lung disease Silica can cause pulmonary complications
Pharmacists	Psyllium dust may cause rhinitis Antibiotic exposure may cause sensitization allergy or contact dermatitis
Printers	Acrylic dyes can cause contact dermatitis and rash

Table 4: Common Workplace Allergens

3.1   Internal and External Air Pollution

Air pollution is a significant global public health problem which seriously threatens the health of communities in both developing and developed countries (Takizawa *et al.*, 2011; Lee, 2013). Smoke released from vehicles in traffic, especially diesel exhaust, and the particles it contains may cause irreversible damage when they enter the respiratory tract. Studies have shown that allergic diseases and asthma are observed with a higher rate in children who live near intensive traffic compared with children who live far from intensive traffic (Gül *et al.*, 2011). Because children breathe in and out at a much higher rate and spend more time in the outdoor air during play and sporting activities, their rate of impact due to air pollution is higher. Diesel exhaust smoke contains ultra small particles that create air pollution, and these have a carrier role for allergenic substances. These particles present the allergenic substances, which adhere to their surfaces, to the immune system and increase the likelihood for the development of an allergy. Ozone is a side-product of diesel exhaust smoke and is an oxidant substance which causes serious damage both to the atmosphere and the respiratory tract of humans. Ozone causes a burn-like inflammation on the surface of the respiratory tract by damaging the inner-layer membrane and this leads to sensitivity. Over time, as the respiratory tract becomes more sensitive, asthma occurs. Symptoms of bronchial narrowing; coughing, wheezing and dyspnea are observed as a result of any external stimulus (smoking, infection, clothing, chemical odors etc). The antioxidants produced by our body can normally overcome low rates of external air pollution. However, when air pollution is increased to a high degree natural antioxidant mechanisms are insufficient, because the burden on the oxidant substance is increased too much and an inflammatory response occurs in the body. This unfavorable response in the body mostly results in recurrent respiratory infections and bronchial asthma. The most efficient way to reverse this picture caused by air pollution is to increase the level of antioxidant substances in the body.

Many asthma patients feel discomfort in cold weather because their respiratory tract has hypersensitivity to the cold. This arises from a cold air allergy. As a result of inhalation of cold air, drying in the throat and narrowing in the trachea occur. In addition, nasal breathing becomes difficult in extremely cold weather. During nasal breathing, there is a sensation of burning and pain. When asthma patients breathe through the mouth, their respiratory tracts become narrowed. The reason for this is that the air entering the mouth has not warmed sufficiently. Nasal breathing has a more relieving effect on the respiratory tract compared with oral breathing, because it enables the air entering the respiratory tract to be warmed and controlled.

The rate of air pollution in closed settings is 2-5 fold higher compared to open settings. In studies performed on this issue, it has been reported that disruption of the internal air quality may lead to various respiratory diseases (asthma etc.), allergic diseases (hypersensitivity pneumonitis etc.) and cancer (Oeder et al., 2012; Gül et al., 2007). Anthropogenic elements including lead, mercury, cadmium, and chrome, among other heavy metals, contaminate the internal air by way of entering/leaking of particles and soil dust from external settings to internal settings. Continuous exposure to low concentrations of volatile organic compounds (VOCs) leads to respiratory tract diseases and asthma. Benzene, toluene, ethyl benzene, xylene and styrene have high toxicities and can be classified as the most harmful VOCs. As the exposure concentration increases, the effects become more severe and coma and mortality may be observed. Strong irritating chemicals are formed as a result of the reaction of internal VOCs with ozone. It has been reported that internal bio-aerosol levels were high in humid and warm regions. Also, VOCs and ozone could reach considerably high levels in areas where smoking, copy devices, printers and computers were present, and indoor use of cleaning materials increased the amount of VOCs at a high rate.

Special attention should be paid to important places like schools and day-care centers because they are closed settings and contain intensive levels of allergens. Classes in schools constitute a high risk in terms of air pollution. Although smoking is generally not permitted and activities including cooking are not performed in schools, high particulate matter (PM) concentrations are observed here. However, it has been proposed that PMs originating from internal settings have a lower toxic effect compared with external PMs because of the chemical composition contained. As a result of the studies performed, it was found that internal air pollution concentrations were at higher levels in crowded settings where there was intensive all-day activity of human groups sensitive to air pollution, including day-care centers and primary schools, especially during winter. Children, whose immune systems are weaker compared with adults, are confronted with allergic diseases in their schools. Tens of students who are in the same area rapidly consume the clean air in the closed setting and share potential risks of asthma and allergies. Chalk dust, newly-painted classes and dust in the classrooms cause allergic diseases. Day-care centers contain more materials that cause allergies in addition to these factors. Day-care centers provide appropriate living areas including carpets, beds, pillows, curtains and hairy toys, all of which have been found to increase the risk of the occurrence of allergic diseases. Preventive measures should absolutely be taken and risk factors should be controlled.

3.2   Mold and Dust Exposure

Mold can be present in both internal and external settings (Gelincik *et al.*, 2005; Jenerowicz, 2012; Reponen, 2013). While mold in external settings can trigger allergies in the spring, summer and autumn, mold in internal settings may cause problems for the whole year. In most cases the harmful effects are due to their toxic effects. In these cases these places should be closet until the reparations are done. It is not always possible but the prolonged exposure makes the symptoms worse.

Any house may produce mold under the appropriate conditions. They may be present even if they cannot be observed visually. Like dust mites, mold also likes humid environments. Mold invades by producing particles which can extend into the air. These particles may transform into house dust. In houses where house dust arising from mold is present, allergy symptoms may be observed if this air is inhaled by a person who has a sensitivity to mold. Formation of mold in internal settings depends on two factors: the first one includes free humidity which occurs as a result of a relative humidity above 50%, and leaks from pipes or plumbing and water sources. The second one is anything on which they can grow. Mold usually grows on wall boards, textile products or wood, but they can grow almost anywhere when they find an appropriate environment.

Dust mites mostly collect in materials including carpets, cushions, pillows and blankets. Dust mite allergy may lead to many symptoms and conditions. These include asthma, difficulty in breathing, coughing, wheezing, a sense of obstruction in the chest, allergic rhinitis, obstructed and draining nose, pruritic and draining eyes, low concentration, headache and sleep disturbances and eczema, pruritus, rash and vesicles in the skin. Dust mite allergy may give continuous discomfort. It has many unfavorable effects on the state of health and quality of life. Children spend a lot of time in their homes. The possibility of asthma in children who grow up in environments that have dust mites is considerably high. The most important treatment method in house dust allergy is keeping away from allergens. Anti-allergen bed sheets, bed clothing and air-cleaning devices are very helpful in keeping away from allergens and creating a treatment opportunity. Further as preventive measures should be emphasized the good cleaning: in all work places, schools, day- care centers and homes. The role of air conditioning is important because in many instances the regular service is neglected, the incoming air in unclean due to unclean tubes and filters.

3.3   Foods

Food allergies and hypersensitivity certain food substances interest many people (Gelincik *et al.*, 2008; Hsu, 2013; Sicherer, 2010). In food allergies, the defense system of the body perceives the proteins found in food substances as dangerous foreign substances and become active. Even the smallest amount of the intolerable food substance may lead to an allergic reaction. Reactions usually occur in a short time following consumption of the food substance and food allergic reactions may be lethal in some cases. In case of an allergy, symptoms usually occur within a few hours following eating. Because the reaction occurs against a protein, purified starch or fat fraction of the food substance in question is tolerated well. The most common symptoms include cutaneous reactions and gastrointestinal symptoms. Anaphylactic shock is an acute allergic reaction which leads to signs in multiple organs. Reactions may be in the form of swelling in the mouth/throat/mucosa, dyspnea, a sense of suffocating, vomiting or loss of consciousness. Allergic shock is severe and severe reactions are frequently observed.

Fruit and vegetable allergies usually arise from cross-allergies. Cross-allergies against fruit and vegetables lead to symptoms in the mouth and throat. Cross-allergy means that the body perceives no difference between the substances against which the body has an allergy and the proteins in other foods, since their proteins are similar. Generally, this condition is manifested with pruritus and swelling in the mouth, nose, lips and throat (oral allergy syndrome). Symptoms also occur in the abdomen/intestines and skin.

Fish allergies may be a severe form of food allergy. Some individuals with a fish allergy have reactions to any kind of fish. Some may show reactions to codfish, but may tolerate salmon, trout or mackerel. Some individuals with fish allergies may give reaction to the steam during fish boiling. Shrimp, crab, crayfish, lobster and other shellfish may lead to allergic and non-allergic reactions. Generally, small amounts taken by foods or steam are sufficient for severe reactions. Since the main allergen found in shellfish sea products is also found in mollusks including snails, calamari and mussels, cross-reactions between different species is common. Mite and cockroach allergies may lead to cross-allergies with shellfish sea products and mollusks, but this usually has no clinical significance.

Pea, soybean, lupine flour and peanuts belong to the same vegetable family. Therefore, cross-reactions may occur between these species. For example, lupine flour may lead to allergic reactions in some individuals with a peanut allergy. Lupine flour is added to some full- and half-cooked cake-pie products. Although peanuts are among the food substances which trigger severe allergic reactions most commonly, not all individuals with a peanut allergy have severe reactions. Although most individuals with a peanut allergy tolerate other tree nuts, it should be noted that these are generally observed together in foods. The person may give a reaction to one or more hazelnut species. Seeds which lead to allergic reactions include sesame seed, sunflower seed and poppy seed. Nut and seed allergies may lead to severe reactions.

In wheat allergies, one or more proteins in wheat, rye and barley may trigger allergic symptoms. Positive allergy tests are generally observed for wheat without a food allergy with wheat intake. Therefore, it is especially important to confirm if only a positive test result is present or not for a clinical allergy or for example hay field pollen allergy. Wheat allergy occurs when people inhale flour, but these people may tolerate foods in which wheat is used. Celiac disease is a chronic inflammatory disease in which wheat gluten, barley and rye-like proteins cause an immune reaction in the intestines. The intestines are normalized with a strict gluten-free diet which should continue for a life time. Celiac disease is generally named as gluten intolerance. In children, feeding with cow's milk may cause a risk of allergy. The most common findings include eczema, urticaria, diarrhea and vomiting. The tests are not positive in all children with a milk allergy. Therefore, when a diagnosis should be made elimination of foods should be performed and the diagnostic test should be repeated. Egg allergy is the second most common allergy in children and as with milk allergy, most children grows out of the allergy as they get older. The tolerance limit varies from person to person, but some individuals are so sensitive that they can show reaction to egg protein residues found in cleaned containers. Both egg white and yolk may lead to an allergic reaction. It is important that in day-care centers and schools the children should have a special diet without being real allergic to the food which should be avoided.

3.4   Latex

Currently, the use of latex is becoming more and more common. It is included in many products we use in our homes and workplaces. High-risk groups include healthcare workers (medicine, dentistry etc.) and workers who work in the manufacturing of latex. Allergies to natural rubber latex (NRL) and occupation-related dermal problems (disinfectants, rubber, metals and detergents) associated with dental products are seen very common among dentists. Latex gloves manufacture workers suffer from occupational asthma that is caused by latex allergy. Latex allergy is present in approximately 1% of the world's population. In addition, latex allergy is observed in 17- to 25% of healthcare workers (Madan 2013; Marcoux, 2013; Pontén, 2013).

Latex allergy is the hypersensitivity to the substance which contains the natural latex core (not synthetic) found in rubber trees (Öztürk *et al.*, 2008). If this hypersensitivity reaches advanced dimensions, the individual's life may be jeopardized. It is very dangerous and disadvantageous to come into contact with products containing latex for individuals with latex allergy. As the degree of contact with such type of products increases, the risk also increases. Individuals with latex allergic may experience cross-reactions to tropical fruits - the so called "Latex-fruit syndrome". The history of the patient should be taken and a latex allergy should be considered even in individuals in whom physical examination reveals the mildest findings. Hypotension, tachycardia, urticaria, flushing in the face, sudden dyspnea, pruritus, abdominal pain, syncope and swelling in the lips are the findings that should be noted. If the patient experiences some kind of respiratory difficulty, though to a mild degree, when he/she puts on gloves or inflates a balloon, a latex allergy should be suspected. Skin tests or blood tests can be performed before the diagnosis of a latex allergy.

As with all allergic diseases, the best treatment method for latex allergy is keeping away from the allergic substances which mean prevention, because as the degree of contact of the person who suffers from latex allergy with this substance increases, his/her complaints will increase accordingly. In a person in whom latex allergy is suspected, antihistamines and drugs containing cortisone should be used before treatment. When a latex allergy develops, there is no known special treatment method. The known therapies for allergic reaction are performed in association with supportive treatment.

3.5   Nickel

Nickel is a basic element which is used in different plates and alloys. The pure form of Nickel is as bright as silver. Nickel is one of the most common metals found in our surroundings. Nickel allergy is a reaction of the body as a result of contact with nickel in a person who has hypersensitivity to this substance (Braga, 2013; Garg 2013; Lidén 2013). Nickel allergy may cause eczema in advanced stages in manufacturing workers. This arises from contact with many substances containing nickel including door handles, taps (excluding stainless steel) and coins. It is mostly contained in imitation jewelry, metal covered pots or pans used in kitchens, shiny door handles, zippers, hairclips, pins, knitting needles, scissors, glasses frames, buttons and coins. In addition, nickel may be found in bleaches, hair dyes and some food substances. There are some foods which contain high amounts of nickel (for example, chocolate, peas, lentils, walnuts, sunflower seeds). When people with a nickel allergy consume such foods, their states may deteriorate and their eczema may get worse. If a person with a nickel allergy comes into contact with this substance, allergic eczema may be observed in any part of his/her body. Eczema, whether newly formed or recurrent, causes vesicles and inflamed wounds on the skin in association with redness and swelling in the skin, when the person comes into contact with the substance against which he/she has an allergy. In chronic contact eczema, severe pruritus is observed in association with drying and cracks on the skin.

It is known that nickel allergy is observed more commonly in women compared to men. The most important reason of this is the valuable materials which women carry on their bodies. Especially jewelry placed on the ears, umbilicus and nose after piercings, are among the main factors which trigger nickel allergy. In this way, the contact of nickel with the skin, and even blood, causes the initiation of some hypersensitivity. After an individual becomes allergic to nickel, it is not possible for them to get rid of it completely. However, he/she may alleviate the effects of this allergy by taking precautions and receiving treatment.

4   Conclusion

Allergy is a very common cause of disease in the general population. Multiple factors can trigger this disease. Occupation and environment are also factors for allergic diseases. Occupational and environmental allergic diseases are one of most important public health problems which interest all countries to a great extent. It is known that approximately 15-25% of the world's population is fighting with this disease. Nowadays when adulthood and childhood diseases are investigated, it is clear that the prevalence of allergic diseases has increased. It has been proposed that these changes are related with the increase in occupational and environmental allergens due to industrialization in recent years.

Occupational and environmental allergic diseases are preventable by appropriate preventative strategies. The most efficient approach for prevention and protection is defining and avoiding the allergen. To this end, the most important step in the diagnosis is a detailed history including the genetic predisposition and exposure of occupational and environmental agents. With some basic environmental measures and even simple hygienic rules protection from an allergy may be provided at certain levels in patients with an allergic physique. In this way, the principle of prevention which is the basic aspect of preventive medicine is adopted with early precautions. It is important to increase the public consciousness on the issue and provoke resources (public, private sector, non-governmental organizations etc.). The beneficial impact of occupational and environmental control may be observed after a short period of time. The importance given to the politics of environmental control including the workplace has started to increase in new prevention strategies for allergic diseases. In this context, physicians, engineers, educators, community leaders, politicians and law enforcement officers have important missions together with patients. Conscious environmental protection will inhibit the progression of allergic diseases and decrease treatment costs which will also provide significant financial resources.

The reason for the recent increase in the prevalence of allergic diseases is still being debated. Detailed molecular studies and studies based on analytic epidemiology are needed to evaluate the pathology of these diseases and the effect of the occupational and environmental exposures on the immune system. Further epidemiologic studies investigating the relations between genetic and environmental factors (for example: chemicals in the workplace; indoor and outdoor air pollution, food preservatives etc.) in sensitive individuals will be helpful to better understand the etiology of the disease.

References

Akinbami, L., Moorman JE., Bailey C et al. (2012). Trends in Asthma Prevalence, Health Care Use, and Mortality in the United States, 2001-2010, NCHS Data Brief No: 94.

Asher, MI, Montefort, S., Björkstén, B., et al. (2006) Worldwide time trends in the prevalence of symptoms of asthma, allergic rhinoconjunctivitis, and eczema in childhood: ISAAC Phases One and Three repeat multicountry cross-sectional surveys. The Lancet, 368: 33–743.

Barnes, C.S., Alexis, N.E., Bernstein, J.A, et al., Cohn, JR. (2013) Allergy Clin Immunol Pract. 2013 Mar; 1(2):137-141. Climate Change and Our Environment: The Effect on Respiratory and Allergic Disease, 1(2):137-141.

Braga M, Quecchia C, Perotta C, et al. (2013). Systemic nickel allergy syndrome: nosologic framework and usefulness of diet regimen for diagnosis. Int J Immunopathol Pharmacol. 2013 Jul-Sep;26(3):707-16.

Carlsten, C., Melén, E. (2012) Air. Air pollution, genetics, and allergy: an update. Curr Opin Allergy Clin Immunol.12(5):455-60.

D'Amato, G., Cecchi L, D'Amato M, Liccardi, G. (2010). Urban air pollution and climate change as environmental risk factors of respiratory allergy: an update. J Investig Allergol Clin Immunol. 20: 95-102.

Dinmeze,l S., Ogus C, Erengin, H., Cilli, A., Ozbudak, O., Ozdemir, T. (2005).The prevalence of asthma, allergic rhinitis, andatopy in Antalya, Turkey. Allergy Asthma Proc., 26:403–409.

Dotterud, CK., Storrø, O., Simpson, MR., Johnsen R., Øien T. (2013). The impact of pre- and postnatal exposures on allergy related diseases in childhood: a controlled multicentre intervention study in primary health care, BMC Public Health, 13:123.

Emri, S., Turnagol, H., Basoglu, S., Bacanlı, S., Guven, G.S., Aslan, D. (2005). Asthma-like symptoms prevalence in five Turkish urban centers. Allergol Immunopathol (Madr) 33:270–276.

Friis, UF., Menné T., Flyvholm, MA, Bonde, JP, Johansen, JD. (2013). Occupational allergic contact dermatitis diagnosed by a systematic stepwise exposure assessment of allergens in the work environment. Contact Dermatitis. Sep;69; 69(3):153-63. doi: 10.1111/cod.12102.

Garg S, Thyssen JP, Uter W, et al., (2013). Nickel allergy following European Union regulation in Denmark, Germany, Italy and the U.K.Br J Dermatol. 2013 Oct; 169(4):854-8.

Gelincik, A., Büyüköztürk, S., Gül, H. et al. (2005). The Effect of İndoor Fungi on the Symptoms of Patients with Allergic Rhinitis in Istanbul, Indoor Built Environ. 14 (5):427-432.

Gelincik, A., Büyüköztürk, S., Gül, H.,et al. (2008). Confirmed Prevalence of Food Allergy and Non-allergic Food Hypersensitivity in a Mediterranean Population. Clinical and Experimental Allergy, 38 (8):1333–1341.

Ghosh, R.E., Cullinan, P., Fishwick, D., et al. (2013). Asthma and occupation in the 1958 birth cohort. Thorax. doi:10.1136/ thoraxjnl-2012-202151.

Greiner AN, Hellings PW, Rotiroti G, Scadding GK (2011): Allergic rhinitis. Lancet, 378(9809):2112–2122.

Gül, H., Gaga, EO., Döğeroğlu, T., Özden, Ö., Ayvaz, Ö., Özel, S., Güngör.G. (2011).Respiratory Health Symptoms among Students Exposed to Different Levels of Air Pollution in a Turkish city. Int. J. Environ. Res. Public Health 8(4):1110-1125.

Gül, H., İşsever, H., Güngör, G. (2007). Occupational and Environmental Risk Factors for the Sick Building Syndrome in Modern Offices in Istanbul: A Cross-Sectional Study, Indoor Built Environ. 16: 47-54.

Hong S, Son DK, Lim WR, Kim SH, Kim H, Yum HY, Kwon H. (2012).The prevalence of atopic dermatitis, asthma, and allergic rhinitis and the comorbidity of allergic diseases in children. Environ Health Toxicol.

Hsu JT, Missmer SA, Young MC(2013). Prenatal food allergen exposures and odds of childhood peanut, tree nut, or sesame seed sensitization. Ann Allergy Asthma Immunol., 111(5):391-6.

Jackson, K.D., Howie, L.D., Akinbami, LJ. (2013).Trends in allergic conditions among children: United States, 1997-2011.NCHS Data Brief, 121:1-8.

Jenerowicz, D., Silny, W., Dańczak-Pazdrowska, A., Polańska, A., Osmola Mańkowska, A., Olek-Hrab, K. (2012). Environmental factors and allergic diseases. Ann Agric Environ Med. 19(3): 475-481.

Kauffmann, F., Demenais, F. (2012) Gene-environment interactions in asthma and allergic diseases: challenges and per-spectives. J Allergy Clin Immunol. 130(6):1229-40.

Kauppi P, Linna M, Martikainen J, Mäkelä MJ, Haahtela T. (2013). Follow-up of the Finnish Asthma Programme 2000-2010: reduction of hospital burden needs risk group rethinking, Thorax. 68(3):292-3.

Kim, KH., Lee, C.S., Jeon, J.M., et al. (2013) Analysis of the association between air pollution and allergic diseases expo-sure from nearby sources of ambient air pollution within elementary school zones in four Korean cities. Environ Sci Pollut Res Int,. 20(7):4831-46.

Kim, K.H., Jahan, S.A., Kabir, E.A. (2013) Review on human health perspective of air pollution with respect to allergies and asthma. Environ Int.59:41, 59:41-52.

Kurt E, Demir AU, Cadirci O, Yildirim H, Ak G, Eser TP. (2010). Occupational exposures as risk factors for asthma and allergic diseases in a Turkish population. Int Arch Occup Environ Health. 84(1):45-52.

Kurt E, Metintas S, Basyigit I et al. (2009). Prevalence and Risk Factors of Allergies in Turkey (PARFAIT): results of a multicentre cross-sectional study in adults. PARFAIT Study of the Turkish Thoracic Society Asthma and Allergy Working GroupEur Respir J,.33(4):724-33.

Lee SY, Chang YS, Cho SH (2013). Allergic diseases and air pollution. Asia Pac Allergy. 3(3):145-54

Le Moual, N., Kauffmann, F., Eisen, EA., et al. (2008).The healthy worker effect in asthma: work may cause asthma, but asthma may also influence work. Am J Respir Cr. Care Med, 177:4–10.

Lidén C. (2013). Nickel allergy following EU regulation - more action is needed. Br J Dermatol. 2013 Oct; 169(4):733.

Madan I, Cullinan P, Ahmed SM. (2013). Occupational management of type I latex allergy Occupational Medicine, 63 (6):395-404.

Matheson, M.C. (2013). Association between latitude and allergic diseases: a longitudinal study from childhood to middle-age. Ann Allergy Asthma Immunol., 110(2):80-85.

Marcoux V, Nosib S, Bi H, Brownbridge B. (2013). Intraoperative myocardial infarction: Kounis syndrome provoked by latex allergy. BMJ Case Rep. 2013 Jan 8;2013. pii: bcr2012007581.

Moorman JE, Akinbami LJ, Bailey CM, et al. (2012) National Surveillance of Asthma: United States, 2001–2010, National Center for Health Statistics. Vital Health Stat 3(35).

Mutius, EV. (2004). Influences in allergy: Epidemiology and the environment, Journal of Allergy and Clinical Immunolo-gy, 113(3):373-379.

Oeder, S., Jörres, R.A., Weichenmeier, I., et al. (2012).Airborne indoor particles from schools are more toxic than outdoor particles. Am J Respir Cell Mol Biol., 47(5):575-82.

Oktaria, V., Dharmage, S.C., Burgess, J.A., et al. (2008). Latex Allergy, a Special Risk for Patients with Chronic Illness and Health Care Workers TAF Prev Med Bull , 7(3):265-268.

Ones U, Akcay A, Tamay Z, Guler N, Zencir M. (2006). Rising trend of asthma prevalence among Turkish schoolchildren (ISAAC phases I and III) Allergy, 61:1448-53.

Pawankar, R., Holgate, ST., Canonica, GW., Lockey, RF.(2011). Allergic disease: A major global public health issue, in The WAO White Book on allergy Printed in the United Kingdom, 2011.

Peden D, Reed CE.(2010). Environmental and occupational allergies. JImmunol 125(Suppl 2):S150–160.

Pleil, J.D., Sobus, J.R, Sheppard, P.R, Ridenour, G, Witten ML. (2012). Strategies for evaluating the environment-public health interaction of long-term latency disease: the quandary of the inconclusive case-control study. Chem Biol In-teract. 2012 Apr 5;196; 196(3):68-78.

Pontén A, Hamnerius N, Bruze M. (2013). Occupational allergic contact dermatitis caused by sterile non-latex protective gloves: clinical investigation and chemical analyses. Contact Dermatitis. 68(2):103-10.

Reponen T, Levin L, Zheng S, Vesper S et al.(2013) Family and home characteristics correlate with mold in homes. Envi-ron Res. 124:67-70.

Sicherer SH, Sampson HA. Food allergy. J Allergy Clin Immunol 2010;125(suppl): S116-25.

Shah R, Grammer LC (2012). Chapter 1: an overview of allergens. Allergy Asthma Proc. 2012 May-Jun;33 Suppl 1:S2-5.

T.C.Ministry of Health, (2009). Sağlık Bakanlığı Temel Sağlık Hizmetleri Genel Müdürlüğü. Türkiye Kronik Hava Yolu Hastalıklarını (Astım - KOAH) Önleme Ve Kontrol Programı (2009 - 2013) Eylem Planı, Ankara, Turkey. Available from: www.saglik.gov.tr/.../1.../turkiye-khh-astimkoah-.

Takizawa, H. (2011). Impact of air pollution on allergic disease. Korean J Intern Medicine, 26: 262-273.

Thong, B.Y.-H., Tan, T.C. (2011). Epidemiology and risk factors for drug allergy. British Journal of Clinical Pharmacology, 71: 684–700.

TUİK, (2013).TurkStat, Turkey's Statistical Yearbook, 2012 Turkish Statistical Institute, Printing Division, Ankara.

Valovirta E. 2011. Book on Respiratory Allergies – Raise Awareness, Relieve the Burden. http://wwwefanetorg/documents/EFABookonRespiratoryAllergiesFINALpdf.

Vandenplas O, Worm M, Cullinan P, Park HS, Wijk RG. Occupational Allergy in The WAO White Book on Allergy, Printed in the United Kingdom, 2011.

Wang DY. (2005). Risk factors of allergic rhinitis: genetic or environmental? Therapeutics and Clinical Risk Management, 1(2) 115– 123.

Warner JO, Kaliner MA, Crisci CD, Del Giacco S, Frew AJ, Liu GH, Maspero J, Moon H-B, Takemasa N, Potter PC, Rosenwasser LJ, Singh AB, Valovirta E, Van Cauwenberge P. Allergy practice worldwide: a report by the World Allergy Organization Specialty and Training Council. Allergy and Clinical Immunology International - World Allergy Organization Journal. 2006; 18:4-10; and International Archives of Allergy and Immunology. 2006; 139(2):166-74.

Wertz DA, Pollack M, Rodgers K, Bohn RL, Sacco P, Sullivan SD. (2010). Impact asthma control on sleep, attendance at work, normal activities, and disease burden. Ann Allergy Asthma Immunol., 105(2):118–123.

Wick JY (2013). Occupational Allergies: Working on It. Pharmacy Times. http://www.pharmacytimes.com/publications /issue/2013/April2013/Occupational-Allergies-Working-On-It.

Wong, G.W., Leung, T.F., Ko, F.W. (2013). Changing prevalence of allergic diseases in the Asia-pacific region. Allergy Asthma Immunol Res., 5(5):251-7.

Yeşillik, S., Öztürk, S. (2013). How Can We Prevent Allergy and Allergic Respiratory Diseases Without Drugs? TAF Prev Med Bull., 12(1): 97-104. (Turkish).

Anaphylaxis: Recent Updates in Diagnosis

Gaurav Singh Tomar

Department of Neuroanesthesiology & Critical care
All India Institute of Medical Sciences, New Delhi, India

1   Introduction

Allergy is a disease of our modern civilized society. One hundred and fifty years ago asthma was considered rare and allergic rhinitis was almost unheard of. Allergies are a family of diseases with complex and differing genetic underlying components that predispose allergy-prone individuals to mount symptoms in response to specific disease, drugs and environmental stimuli and pollution. Allergy is defined as 'a hypersensitivity reaction initiated by immunologic mechanisms' which can be either antibody or cell mediated. In other words, allergic individuals have symptoms of asthma, rhinoconjunctivitis, or eczema. The antibody isotype most commonly responsible for allergic reactions is IgE. However, it is important to recognize that not all hypersensitivity reactions that appear to be allergic in nature are necessarily caused by IgE. Approximately 40% of the population has raised IgE levels, while in only 20% are there symptoms of allergy (Cockcroft & Davis 2009; Eckman & Saini, 2009). For example, systemic reactions to dextran, although they mimic anaphylaxis, result from IgG immune complexes. Other allergic reactions seem not to be mediated by antibodies at all. For instance, the pathogenesis of allergic contact dermatitis is attributed to activated antigen-specific lymphocytes. In this chapter, the importance of history taking and tryptase quantification are emphasized. Specific confirmatory diagnostic procedures are organized on the basis of the major causes of perioperative anaphylactic reactions.

2   Allergy History

Before taking an allergy history, adopting a professional but friendly manner, the early establishment of eye contact, and the avoidance of extraneous distractions by interviewers should put patients at their ease. The history need not be time consuming, although patients should be allowed to give their own accounts of symptoms followed by structured prompts or questions.

2.1   The patient's Personal history

Obtaining an accurate patient history is crucial in diagnosing allergic disease. Initially, patients should be allowed to give their own account of symptoms followed by structured prompts or questions to cover the given points. Listen to the patient's account of the symptoms. Patients often have their own way of describing symptoms. Some disease-related symptoms are:

Allergic rhinitis
Nasal congestion; rhinorrhoea; sneezing; itching
Asthma
Wheezing; dyspnoea; chest tightness; cough
Anaphylaxis
Flushing; urticaria; pruritus of lips, tongue, palms, and soles; gastrointestinal cramping, nausea, vomiting, and diarrhoea; dyspnoea, chest tightness and wheezing; palpitations, tachycardia and chest pain; syncope or near syncope, altered mental status or dizziness; uterine contractions in women.

Table 1: Symptoms of different allergic conditions

2.2 Frequency and Severity of the Symptoms

Establish whether there is a personal or family history of asthma, rhinitis, and eczema. If one parent has allergic disease, then there is an approximate 40% likelihood that each of the offspring will have symptoms of allergy. If both parents have allergic disease, then the likelihood that a child has an allergic condition increases to roughly 80–85% (Cockcroft & Davis 2009). Ask whether the symptoms are seasonal or perennial. Symptoms of aero allergen-induced rhinitis and asthma may be seasonal if caused by trees, grasses, weeds, or moulds. It is helpful for the evaluating physician to understand the general timing of the pollen seasons in the community in which the patient lives.

The clinical manifestation of these reactions is not infrequently an almost immediate generalized response with bronchospasm and hypotension. The degree of severity varies and does not allow differentiation between an IgE-mediated or non-IgE mediated reaction resulting from nonspecific mediator release. In most cases, perioperative anaphylaxis is characterized by severe respiratory and cardiovascular manifestations such as arterial hypotension and cardiovascular collapse. The mortality from these reactions is in the range from 3 to 6%, and an additional 2% of patients experience significant residual brain damage.

2.3 Onset of Symptoms

Clinical signs and symptoms of anaesthetic anaphylaxis usually start within 5–10 min after intravenous administration of the responsible agent but can occur within seconds. In contrast, anaphylaxis from natural rubber latex (NRL) and antiseptics exhibit a more delayed onset and generally occurs during maintenance anaesthesia or recovery, as a result of later application or absorption through skin, mucosal surfaces and/or soft tissues, or removal of a tourniquet. In patients allergic to latex, bronchospasm may also be observed early following arrival of a sensitized patient in the operating theatre. Anaphylaxis from colloids can occur immediately or demonstrate a more delayed onset. Careful retrospective assessment of medical history and revision of records from local and/or generalized anaesthesia has been demonstrated to reveal symptoms and signs suggestive for the patient being at risk for perioperative anaphylaxis. For example, in a series (Mertes *et al.*, 2003) on 30 latex allergic patients (34%), careful revision of medical history performed after the reaction revealed symptoms highly suggestive for latex allergy, already to be present before the reaction. This strongly reinforces the need for an active policy to identify patients at risk during the pre-anaesthetic visit.

3 Co-existing Conditions

Identification of particular underlying conditions can also help to identify the causative compound(s). Atopic individuals are particularly at risk for anaphylaxis from NRL during anaesthesia. Patients with mastocytosis are prone to develop perioperative anaphylactic-like reactions and patients with C1-esterase inhibitor deficiency may experience an exacerbation of their disease with cutaneous, laryngeal, or gastrointestinal swellings.

4   Diagnosis

Diagnosis of drug induced anaphylaxis is usually straightforward. Sometimes, it can be hampered as a broad spectrum of different drugs can elicit heterogeneous allergic and nonallergic reactions with distinct and sometimes unclear pathological mechanisms. Problems are certainly compounded as multiple drugs need to be administered during general anaesthesia in particular. In addition, nonanaesthesia related drugs or procedures (e.g. disinfection) are sometimes administered / performed in the perioperative period and can also be the cause of an allergic reaction. Correct management of anaphylaxis especially during anaesthesia requires a multidisciplinary approach with prompt recognition and treatment of the acute event by the attending anaesthesiologist, and subsequent determination of the responsible agent(s) with strict avoidance of subsequent administration of all incriminated and/or cross-reacting compounds. However, correct identification of the causative compound(s) and safe alternatives is not always straightforward and, too often, not done.

This chapter is not intended to discuss acute management of anaesthesia-related anaphylaxis but summarizes the major causes of anaphylaxis during anaesthesia and the diagnostic approach of this rare but potentially life threatening complication. Apart from general principles about the diagnostic approach, history taking and importance of tryptase quantification, more specific confirmatory diagnostic procedures are organized on the basis of the major causes of perioperative anaphylactic reactions. The problem in the assessment of the reliability of tests is that, when a single diagnostic test is negative, it is impossible to determine whether it is a false-negative test or whether the patient is tolerant to the tested agent, unless the agent is administered. Ideally, diagnosis of anaphylaxis during anaesthesia should rest upon different confirmatory tests, rather than on a single one. In the event of discrepancies between different tests, an alternative compound that tested completely negative is advocated. In order to reduce the risk for false-negative results, the diagnostic approach of anaesthetic anaphylaxis is best postponed until 4–6 weeks after the acute event, because of refractoriness of the effector cell or temporarily depletion of specific IgE (sIgE) antibodies. Alternatively, sensitivity of skin tests might decrease over time, a phenomenon particularly relevant for antibiotics. In contrast, skin tests for neuromuscular blocking agent (NMBA) will usually remain positive for a long period of time. Results may merely cause an inconvenience (unnecessary avoidance of a safe drug), whereas false-negative or equivocal results may be extremely dangerous and severely undermine correct secondary prevention.

4.1   Clinical and Laboratory Evaluation of Allergy

Treatment for allergic diseases is often initiated based on the patient's history alone. Symptoms of type I hypersensitivity that begin after a clearly defined environmental exposure should prompt institution of environmental controls to eliminate future exposure to the suspected allergen. Pharmacotherapy may also be started if environmental controls are not able to eliminate the allergen to levels that do not precipitate symptoms. However, many patients will continue to have symptoms despite these initial therapeutic maneuvers. In such cases, the allergen may not have been correctly identified by history, prompting a more comprehensive search to identify the relevant allergen to institute more aggressive and definitive environmental controls. In other instances, pharmacotherapy may either not be providing sufficient relief from the symptoms, or side effects or toxicity may be limiting the use of these agents. In these cases, testing to confirm that allergic disease is indeed causing the patient's symptoms is important to reassure the patient and physician that the therapeutic plan is indeed on target to mitigate the patient's suffering, and whether pharmacotherapy should be continued or increased. In cases where the maximal pharmacological therapy that the patient desires or can tolerate has been reached, then allergen testing is critical to decide whether specific immunotherapy or anti-IgE therapy should be considered. This chapter reviews the *in vivo* and in vitro tests that have evidence-based utility in allergic disease diagnosis, as well as tests that are used by some practitioners in diagnosing allergy, but have unproven effectiveness.

4.1.1 Serum/plasma tryptases (Mast cell tryptase)

Tryptase is a mast cell tetrameric neutral serine protease that consists out of two major forms, i.e. a & b-tryptase that share approximately 90% of sequence homology. The measurement of serum tryptase is used to diagnosis conditions where mast cell activation occurs either acutely, such as in anaphylaxis, or in situations of ongoing mast cell activation, such as in systemic mastocytosis (Caughey, 2006). Mast cells contain approximately 300–700 times more tryptase than do basophils, and consequently serum tryptase is more reflective of a mast cell source. There are two forms of mast-cell-derived tryptase: α-tryptase and β-tryptase. The concentration of serum α-tryptase is considered to be reflective of the number of mast cells, while serum β-tryptase is a marker of mast cell activation. Pro-b-tryptase is secreted constitutively and serves as a measure for mast cell number, whereas mature-b-tryptase rather reflects mast cell activation. Human basophils also contain tryptase, but their levels are 300 to 700 folds lower than in skin or lung mast cells. An elevated total serum tryptase level (pro-b and pro-a and mature-b tryptase) is therefore highly indicative for mast cell degranulation, as seen in systemic anaphylaxis. (Caughey, 2006).

Levels of α-tryptase are obtained by subtracting the concentration of β-tryptase from the total tryptase concentration. In healthy subjects, total serum tryptase levels range between 1 and 10 ng/mL while serum β-tryptase levels are less than 1 ng/mL. In contrast, if baseline serum total tryptase levels are greater than 20 ng/mL and serum β-tryptase levels are greater than 1 ng/mL, systemic mastocytosis should be strongly considered. If an anaphylactic event is suspected, blood for total and β-tryptase should be obtained from 30 minutes to 4 hours after the episode occurs. Although because of ethnic differences there is no absolute cut-off level for diagnosing anaphylaxis, levels above 12–14 ng/mL are generally accepted as indicative of anaphylaxis. A rise in total tryptase can be quantified in serum (or plasma) as soon as 30 min after onset of symptoms, but sampling is recommended 60–120 min after onset-of symptoms. Tryptase's half-life is about 120 min, and levels gradually decrease over time (Laroche, 1991). To enable comparison with baseline levels, a new sample should be collected >2 days after the reaction. Tryptase levels may remain elevated in cases of late-onset, biphasic or protracted cell activation and in association with an underlying mastocytosis (Schwartz *et al.*, 1987; Schwartz *et al.*, 1995) Discrimination between mature b tryptase and total serum tryptase is not only likely to result in greater specificity in the diagnosis of anaphylaxis but can also be helpful when anaphylaxis occurs in the setting of mastocytosis (Edston & Hage-Hamsten, 1998). False-negative results have been attributed to a mechanism where the reaction involves basophils rather than mast cells, whereas false positive results have been reported in cases of extreme stress such as hypoxemia and major trauma. Serum tryptase does not differentiate between immunological and non-immunological mast cell activation, and does not contribute in the identification of the causative compound(s). However, in non-immunological reactions rise of tryptase is less prevalent and usually less pronounced than in immunological mast cell activation (Fisher & Baldo, 1998).

4.1.2   IgE Level

The core of the allergic response lies in the quantity and specificity of IgE production of patients to allergens. IgE levels are low in the fetus and newborn because these molecules do not readily cross the placenta. In general, serum IgE increases with age until the first half of the second decade of life, whereupon they begin to decrease proportionately with age. Therefore, it is important to examine total IgE levels in the framework of age-adjusted reference values for non-allergic persons. Allowing for these caveats, measuring total IgE can be useful as shown by the fact that total serum IgE >100 IU/mL before age of 6 years is a well-recognized risk factor for allergic rhinitis (Hamilton, 2010).

However, it must also be emphasized that the presence or absence of IgE antibodies alone is not conclusive of disease. For example, smokers often have high IgE levels in the absence of demonstrable allergic disease. Therefore, IgE levels may be used only as supportive information in the diagnosis of allergy and not in isolation. Testing for allergen-specific IgE may be done in two ways: *in vivo* tests such as skin testing and in vitro measurement in blood samples. In general, skin testing tends to be more sensitive whereas allergen-specific IgE measurements in vitro may be more specific. Skin testing is usually performed first for evaluation of sensitization to aeroallergens. However, there are other instances, such as in evaluation of sensitivity to hymenoptera, where determination of allergen-specific IgE can be an important adjunct to skin testing, especially when skin-testing results are negative. Both skin testing and in vitro determination of allergen-specific IgE are generally used before direct allergen provocation as this testing has the risk of inciting significant allergic reactions. (Joint Task Force on Practice Parameters, 2008).

4.1.3   Lung Function Tests

Peak flow monitoring and spirometry, together with an assessment of reversibility (either before or after a bronchodilator), or repeated peak flow measurements at home in order to detect diurnal variation, will confirm or exclude the reversibility of airflow obstruction (i.e. asthma) in the majority of cases. Measurements of airway hyper-responsiveness by means of histamine or methacholine inhalation testing may be helpful, particularly in mild cases where lung function may be normal and response to a bronchodilator is absent. In these circumstances, a low-histamine PC20 [i.e. a provocation concentration that causes a 20% reduction in FEV1 (forced expiratory volume in 1 second)] within the asthmatic range (less than 8 mg/mL) would confirm the need for a trial of bronchodilator therapy and further peak flow monitoring.

4.1.4   Skin Prick Test [SPT] & Intradermal Test [IDT]

Skin testing can take one of two forms: epicutaneous (more usually known as skin prick testing, or SPT) or intradermal testing (IDT). Skin prick testing usually has sufficient sensitivity and specificity to be the sole method of skin testing necessary for most clinical scenarios. In allergic rhinitis, the sensitivity of SPT is 85–87% and its specificity 79–86%, while in allergic asthma the sensitivity of SPT has been reported to be as high as 91–98%.(Brockow, 2002) There are some situations, however, such as testing for penicillin allergy or venom hypersensitivity, in which intradermal testing is warranted because of its increased sensitivity.

Skin prick tests are usually performed either on the volar aspect of the patient's forearm or on the back. Whereas the back is considered to be more reactive, the forearm is more convenient. A drop of an allergen extract is placed on a previously cleaned area of skin surface; a sharp instrument, either a needle or a lancet, is then passed through the extract drop at a 45° to 60° angle to the skin and the skin is lifted gently to create a small break in the epidermis to enable allergen penetration into the skin. Test sites, which should be 2–2.5 cm apart to avoid overlapping reactions from occurring, should be marked for allergen identification and the excess allergen extract carefully wiped away to avoid contamination with other test sites. For routine clinical use, wheal size should be measured at 15–20 minutes and recorded as the mean of the longest diameter and the orthogonal diameter (i.e. the diameter at 90° to the midpoint of the longest diameter, excluding pseudopodia).

SPT are considered positive when the wheal and flare reaction exceeds 3/3 mm. IDT are performed by injecting 0.05 ml into the dermis of the forearm or back through a hypodermic needle. Reactions are read after 20 min. The IDT is considered positive if the diameter of the obtained wheal exceeds 8 mm and doubles with respect to the injection bleb. The choice of tests can therefore be based on other factors such as age of the patients (SPT being less painful and thus more suitable for children), cost, and ease of performance. IDT is usually restricted to patients with negative or equivocal SPT results. Although highly reliable, these skin tests do not demonstrate absolute diagnostic accuracy. (Fisher & Bowey, 1997).

	False negative skin test	False positive skin test
Etiology:	When patient on antihistaminics (H-1 blocker), or a drug with antihistaminic properties ex. tricyclic antidepressant (TCA) before skin testing.	If the skin test extract unknowingly contains histamine or causes an irritant reaction. ex. dermographism (in 2–5% of the population)
Diagnosis:	A positive control with histamine (10 mg/mL) should be used at one skin-testing site.	A drop of saline or vehicle instead of allergen extract used at one skin-testing site.

*To be deemed as positive, allergen-induced wheals should have a maximum diameter at least 3 mm greater than the appropriate negative control.

Table 2: False negative & positive skin tests

There are specific circumstances regarding skin test that deserve special notice, particularly anaphylaxis and food allergy. Following anaphylaxis, skin testing should be delayed for at least 4 weeks as testing following may give a false negative result to the allergen that actually caused the anaphylactic episode. This situation often arises in situations where anaphylaxis has occurred to foods, insect venom, or drugs. Investigation of possible allergic reactions to food also warrants special mention as extensive research has been performed in this field that has been further evaluated by double-blind, placebo-controlled food challenges. Such studies reveal that a negative skin prick test has a negative predicative accuracy of greater than 90%, essentially ruling out an IgE-mediated reaction to the food being tested. (Thong & Yeow, 2004).

Finally, skin testing should not be performed in the absence of a clinical history suggesting a particular drug/food allergy because a positive skin test may reveal the presence of allergen-specific IgE, but may not mean the patient is allergic to the drug/agent giving the positive skin test. Similarly, testing to venom in the absence of a positive history is not recommended because it is estimated that one-quarter of people without history of systemic reaction may have positive skin tests to these allergen extracts. Although highly reliable, these skin tests do not demonstrate absolute diagnostic accuracy. (Fisher *et al.*, 1999; Fisher & Baldo, 2000).

4.1.5 *In vitro* Laboratory Tests

In vitro measurement of allergen-specific IgE is the laboratory equivalent of clinical skin testing. Although there is some variation among different proprietary methods for measurement of allergen-specific IgE, the basic concept is that an allergen is linked to a solid phase to which a patient's serum is added. With incubation, the patient's allergen-specific IgE binds to the allergen-linked solid phase. After washing of unbound patient antibody from the allergen-linked solid phase, a labeled human anti-IgE antibody is added; this will then bind to the patient's IgE that is bound to the allergen-linked solid phase. Detection of this human anti-IgE antibody bound to the patient's allergen-specific IgE provides the readout for this assay. It is important to note that, although this general scheme is used to detect allergen specific IgE, there are substantial differences among the manufacturers of these assays, which does not allow for complete interchangeability of results. For instance, these differences include variations in the different solid phases to which allergen is bound, as well as in the composition, concentration, and potency of the specific allergen linked to the solid phase. Variations in the allergen used result in different populations of a patient's IgE that are detected in the assay. (Florvaag *et al.*, 2005; Gueant, 1991).

More recently the advent of chip technology has improved allergen-specific IgE detection, as a single chip is able to identify multiple allergens in as little as 20 µL of serum. This system has the major benefit of allowing the recognition of cross-reactivity of a patient's IgE against structurally similar antigens from different sources. This test is currently available in Europe only. Just as in skin testing, where the size of the test corresponds to the likelihood that a patient has allergy to that allergen but does not reflect the severity of the clinical reaction.

4.1.6 Basophil Histamine Release Test

Allergy screening may also be performed by assessing histamine released from blood basophils after the addition of allergen extract. In this test, blood samples, which may be as small as 20 µL for each allergen, are pipetted into the wells of an ELISA plate precoated with the suspected allergens. The plate is then incubated at 37°C for up to 1 hour and the resultant histamine release estimated. Basophil histamine release, which is usually performed by specialist laboratories, takes only a few hours to perform. This test is semi quantified on the basis of the concentration of the allergen extract that gives rise to a certain amount of histamine released. As the basophils of about 5% of the population do not release histamine in vitro, a positive response to anti-IgE, used as a positive control, is absolutely necessary to validate a negative result. Furthermore, as the majority of the population has some circulating IgE, a positive result to anti-IgE is not indicative of the presence of allergy in the absence of a corroborative history. (Abuaf *et al.*, 1999; Ebo *et al.*, 2002; Torres *et al.*, 2004).

A second use of the basophil degranulation test is in the investigation of chronic spontaneous urticaria. At least 30% of patients with this condition have histamine releasing auto-antibodies directed to either IgE or FcεR1, the high-affinity receptor for IgE. Evidence for these antibodies comes from *in vivo* studies of autoreactivity with the autologous serum skin test (ASST) in which autologous intradermal injection of serum causes a wheal and flare response. In vitro detection of these antibodies is performed by incubation of 40 µl of patient's serum with white blood cells, containing 1–2% basophils, from a healthy non-atopic donor for 1 hour in the presence of IL-3.

4.1.7 *In vivo* Provocation Tests

The clinical history may occasionally not provide a clear diagnosis, such as when a patient's shortness of breath has some but not all of the features of asthma. Additionally, there will be instances when the clinical history of manifestations of allergic disease does not match skin testing or *in vitro* assays assessing antigen-specific IgE. In these situations, *in vivo* provocation testing can be considered to assess further the relationship between symptoms and physiological end points. Such tests may use pharmacological agents and therefore not be allergen specific, for instance inhaled methacholine or histamine challenges used in asthma assessment.

Organ challenge tests can be performed to assess whether or not a specific allergen is definitively causing a specific constellation of symptoms suggestive of an allergic reaction. The site of organ challenge is based on the patient's history and may include the conjunctiva, upper or lower respiratory tract, or skin for allergic contact dermatitis or insect sting. These tests are usually reserved for the situation where skin test or *in vitro* allergen IgE results do not correspond to patient history or clinical situation. Most often, these tests are performed in a controlled research setting because of the possible risk of severe, life-threatening reactions to direct organ allergen challenge.(Bernstein *et al.*, 2008)

4.2 Allergy Diagnosis in Relation with its Etiology

4.2.1 Systemic Mastocytosis

Patients with mastocytosis may have elevated levels of baseline total serum tryptase (between episodes). However, it should be noted that both mastocytosis and mast-cell-activating syndromes can be present with normal baseline serum tryptase levels. Tryptase levels obtained during an asymptomatic phase are a reasonably good screening test to diagnose episodes due to underlying systemic mastocytosis. (Schwartz *et al.*, 1995)

An elevated tryptase level above 20 ng/mL is highly specific, but again this test lacks sensitivity, and a normal baseline level does not rule out the presence of mastocytosis.(Jogie-Brahim *et al.*,2004) Also, the majority of patients suffering from mastocytosis have a point mutation in the c-kit receptor (D816V), which can be demonstrated in bone marrow. A test for D816V on blood is now available, but this appears to be less sensitive than the same test performed on the bone marrow. It should also be remembered that elevated total serum tryptase can occur in myeloproliferative disorders, the hypereosinophilic syndrome associated with FIP1L1/PDGFRA mutations, and end-stage kidney disease.

4.2.2 Hereditary Angioedema (HAE)

Recognizing HAE is often difficult due to the wide variability in disease expression. This disease may be similar in its presentation to other forms of angioedema resulting from allergies or other medical conditions, but it is significantly different in cause and treatment. When hereditary angioedema is misdiagnosed as an allergy it is most commonly treated with steroids and epinephrine, drugs that are usually ineffective in treating a hereditary angioedema episode. Other misdiagnoses have resulted in unnecessary exploratory surgery for patients with abdominal swelling and other hereditary angioedema patients report that their abdominal pain was wrongly diagnosed as psychosomatic. HAE accounts for only a small fraction of all cases of angioedema. To avoid potentially fatal consequences such as upper airway obstruction and unnecessary abdominal surgery, the importance of a correct diagnosis cannot be over-emphasized. (Bhivgade, 2012) A blood test, ideally taken during an episode, can be used to diagnose the condition.

Analysis of complement C1 inhibitor levels may play a role in diagnosis. C4 and C2 are complementary components.

4.2.3   Blood Components and IgA Deficiency

The presence of anti-IgA in an IgA deficient recipient is a possible cause of anaphylactic transfusion reactions. Approximately 20% of anaphylactic transfusion reactions in a Caucasian population may be associated with anti-IgA in IgA deficient recipients. Ideally, investigation would be done to determine if anti-IgA antibodies are present and for the transfusion of various blood components, it should be harvested from IgA deficient donors. If the patient is not IgA deficient and no anti-IgA has been detected, and the patient has experienced only a single anaphylactic or anaphylactoid reaction, a trial transfusion of unwashed blood components may be performed under controlled conditions, including patient consent, premedication, and close medical supervision. If an anaphylactic reaction occurs again, the patient should be transfused using washed components. (Um *et al.*, 2013 & Singh *et al.*, 2014)

4.2.4   Drugs and related Compounds

Many of these drugs can elicit adverse drug reactions that fall apart into two major types. First, reactions that is usually dose-dependent and related to the pharmacological properties of the drug and/or its metabolites. Second, reactions that are unrelated to the drug's pharmacological characteristics and that are less dose-dependent. These reactions comprise drug intolerance, idiosyncratic reactions and drug-induced immune-mediated allergic and nonimmune-mediated so-called pseudo-allergic or anaphylactoid reactions. Allergy to NMBAs, latex and antibiotics are the most frequent substances involved, allergy to other substances are by far less frequent.

Neuromuscular blocking agents

Cross-reactivity between NMBA is said to be common because of ubiquitous ammonium groups in these drugs. The estimated prevalence of cross-reactivity between NMBA is about 65% by skin tests and 80% by radioimmuno assay (RIA) inhibition tests. [27] While some pairings are common, the patterns of cross-reactivity vary considerably between patients. It is unusual that an individual is allergic to all NMBA. Cross-reactivity depends on the configuration of the paratope of the antibody, which might either completely correspond to the ammonium epitope or extend to an adjacent part of the NMBA molecule, to the structure of the NMBA (flexibility, inter-ammonium distance) and to the relative affinities of the different NMBA for their sIgE antibodies. However, it must be kept in mind that some patients might suffer from multiple allergies. For a comprehensive comparison between SPT and IDT for NMBA, there is no significant difference in the reliability of diagnostic yield of SPT and IDT. (Levy, 2000) There are currently no NMBA-specific IgE assays readily available, except for suxamethonium (Phadia c202). Unfortunately, on several occasions, sIgE for suxamethonium has been reported to be too insensitive (sensitivity 30–60%). Different authors have proposed to use a quaternary ammonium (choline chloride), a p-amino phenyl phosphoryl-choline, or morphine-based solid phase sIgE assay in preference to different NMBA-specific IgE assays to assess sensitization from quaternary ammonium determinants of NMBA. In several of these studies, the assays proved to be highly efficient with sensitivity and specificity approximating or exceeding 90%. (Berg CM *et al.*, 2003; Dhonneur *et al.*, 2004; Fisher, 2004).

Cross-reactivity and identification of a safe alternative should primarily be asserted by skin tests, but functional assays such as histamine release tests or flow-assisted analysis of *in vitro* activated basophils can provide valuable adjuncts. Evidence has accumulated that flow cytometric analysis and quantification of *in vitro* activated basophils can add to the diagnosis of anaphylaxis from NMBA. In these series, sensitivity and specificity of the technique is around 60 and 90% respectively (Berg CM *et al.*, 2003; Fisher, 2004). In a study sensitivity of the basophil activation assay for rocuronium was 92%, whereas specificity was 100% (Dhonneur et al., 2004). In addition, the technique proved clearly complementary to skin tests in the assessment of cross-reactivity and identification of a safe alternative. Larger comprehensive studies are required to confirm these data and allow the technique to enter mainstream diagnostic approach. A systematic preoperative screening for the potential of anaphylaxis from NMBA is not recommended.

Natural rubber latex (NRL)

In most patients, diagnosis of NRL anaphylaxis can readily be established by quantification of sIgE (k82), skin tests, or both. Although these tests are highly reliable, results of are not always unequivocal, and some patients might need additional tests such as basophil activation or challenge tests to establish diagnosis. (Tamayo *et al.*, 2006; Hepner & Castells 2003).

Antibiotics

The diagnostic approach for allergic reactions to (b-lactam antibiotics have recently been standardized under the aegis of ENDA, the EAACI interest group on drug hypersensitivity. Skin tests start with SPT, which are, if negative, followed by IDT. Skin testing should not be limited to the classical and commercial reagents benzylpenicilloyl poly-l-lysine (PPL) and so-called minor determinants mixture (MDM), but should include amoxicillin (AX) and ampicillin (AMP), as well as the culprit compound(s). *In vitro* assays to quantify sIgE for several penicillin determinants (Phadia penicilloyl G (c1), penicilloyl V (c2), amoxycilloyl (c6), ampicilloyl (c5) and cefaclor (c7)) are available and, although generally less sensitive than skin tests, constitute a valuable and safe tool in the diagnostic approach for patients with suspected IgE mediated b-lactam allergy. In a comparison between quantification of sIgE and basophilic CD63 expression, in 58 patients suffering from skin test-proven b-lactam allergy and 30 healthy control individuals, sensitivity and specificity of the assays approximated 38% and 87% for sIgE and 50% and 94% for the basophil activation test respectively. (Sanz *et al.*, 1996).

Provocation tests with b-lactam antibiotics should be restricted to those patients with a suggestive history and negative IgE and skin test investigations. Vancomycin can elicit two types of immediate hypersensitivity reactions; the red man syndrome and anaphylaxis. The red man syndrome typically consists of pruritus, burning sensation, an erythematous eruption that spreads over face, neck and upper torso. Less frequently angio-oedema, dyspnoea and hypotension can occur. Signs generally appear within 5–10 min after start of infusion and are often associated with too rapid (<1 h) infusion of the first dose and result from nonspecific mediator release from mast cells and basophils. Teicoplanin can also cause red man syndrome. Documented cases of IgE-mediated allergy from vancomycin remain anecdotal. Original intradermal test with vancomycin should be performed below a concentration of 10 lg/ml. (Khurana & De Belder, 1999).

Quinolones constitute the third most important group of antibiotics involved in perioperative anaphylaxis. Unlike penicillin, there are no validated skin testing reagents and readily available sIgE assays to aid in confirming the presence of sIgE antibodies to vancomycin and quinolones. Skin tests with quinolones are not reliable, as these drugs can induce direct histamine release (Scherer & Bircher, 2005). It should also be emphasized that antibiotics such as bacitracin and rifamycin, applied locally to irrigate wounds, can also elicit potentially life-threatening anaphylaxis and must not be overlooked. Anaphylactic reactions from locally applied antibiotics have been reported after removal of tourniquet.

Hypnotics

Diagnosis of anaphylaxis from thiopental generally rests upon skin tests and/or quantification of sIgE that is available for research purposes. As for most other hypnotics SPT are performed with undiluted drug, whereas for IDT 0.05 ml of a 10- to 100-fold dilution of the commercially stock solution is tested. Thiopental sodium may show cross reactivity with barbiturate analogues such as pentobarbitone, phenobarbitone and methohexital (Marone & Stellato, 1992). Methohexital is a barbiturate derivative generally applied for brief surgical procedures and rarely induces anaphylaxis. Although their frequent application, anaphylaxis from nonbarbiturate hypnotics is rare. Propofol (2-6 di-isopropylphenol) is an alkyl phenol that bears two isopropyl groups that may act as antigenic epitopes. There is one report on allergy from propofol that emphasis the drug should be omitted in patients with allergy from eggs or soy, from which lecithins are present in the propofol vehicle. However, up to now we did not observe anaphylaxis from propofol in patients with egg or soy allergy. According to sIgE data, it has been postulated that propofol is contraindicated in patients with anaphylaxis from NMBA. This is, however, not the experience of others. Actually, in analogy with allergy for thiopental sodium, patients with propofol allergy can demonstrate clinically irrelevant IgE antibodies against NMBA. Diagnosis of propofol allergy has been established by skin tests, sIgE and histamine-release tests. Alternatively, propofol has been demonstrated to induce a concentration-dependent histamine release from human lung mast cells and can elicit bronchospasm at higher doses. Anaphylaxis from etomidate, an imidazole derivative, that is structurally unrelated to any of the other intravenous hypnotics and ketamine, a phenylcyclidine derivative, is extremely rare. Midazolam hydrochloride is a short-acting imidazo benzodiazepine that rarely causes anaphylaxis. In those series, diagnosis of midazolam anaphylaxis was established upon SPT with undiluted drug and IDT (Marone & Stellato, 1992; Karila *et al.*, 2006).

Opioids

Generalized reactions to opioids [e.g. morphine, codeine] and synthetic opioids such as meperidine (pethidine) usually result from nonspecific mast cell activation, rather than from IgE-mediated degranulation. Particularly, skin mast cells are sensitive to nonspecific activation by opioids. In contrast, mast cells of the heart, lung and gastrointestinal system as well as basophils are not sensitive to opioids. As a consequence, most of these reactions are not life-threatening and include pruritus, urticaria and mild hypotension but are frequently misinterpreted as drug allergy. Fentanyl appears not to induce nonspecific mediator release from mast cells. Evidence for IgE-mediated reactions from opioids in the literature is restricted to some case reports on anaphylaxis from fentanyl (Tomar *et al.*, 2012), meperidine, codeine, morphine and pholcodine. None of these cases reports on potential cross-reactivity between the different opioid subclasses phenanthrenes (e.g. morphine, codeine), phenylpiperedines (alfentanyl, fentanyl, remifentanyl, sufentanyl and meperidine) and diphenylheptanes (methadone and propoxyphene). Therefore, historically, the recommendation has been to switch to a different subclass with a distinct chemical structure in order to avoid antibody recognition. However, the observation that codeine, meperidine and methadone, representatives of the different opioid subclasses react with morphine antibodies put into question this practice. In the absence of validated drug specific diagnostic tools, correct diagnosis of opiate allergy remains a clinical challenge. Particularly, because SPT have been demonstrated to be not useful for this purpose and morphine sIgE, as addressed above, does not per se indicate sensitization from this drug, but might rather mirror sensitization from quaternary ammonium structures from NMBA. Placebo controlled challenges may be required to diagnose opioid allergy.

Aspirin and other NSAIDS

During the last two decades, evidence has emerged that bronchospasm and urticaria/angio-oedema from these drugs result from inhibition of cyclooxygenase (COX)-1 iso-enzyme with subsequent depletion of prostaglandin E2 and unrestrained synthesis of cysteinyl leukotrienes (cys-LT) and release of mediators from mast cells and eosinophil's. Weak COX-1 inhibitors, such as paracetamol and partial inhibitors of both COX-1 and COX-2, such as nimesulide and meloxicam, can cross-react but generally only at high drug doses (Pierzchalska et al., 2000). Selective COX-2 inhibitors do rarely precipitate asthma and/or urticaria/angio-oedema and are generally (but not always) well tolerated. Alternatively, all NSAIDs, including the selective COX-2 inhibitors, can induce urticaria or anaphylaxis. Currently, diagnosis of ASA and NSAID-induced hypersensitivity reactions can only be established by drug provocation tests. There are currently no sIgE assays for ASA or NSAID available. The diagnostic value of histamine and cys-LT release assays and flow-assisted quantification of *in vitro* activated basophils remains to be established. (Gamboa *et al.*, 2004; Gamboa *et al.*, 2003; Lebel *et al.*, 2001) In our department patients with hypersensitivity reactions from ASA and NSAID are challenged with incremental doses of a selective COX-2 inhibitor, and some positive provocations have been observed. Acetaminophen (paracetamol) is an extensively used analgesic and antipyretic that was perioperatively frequently administered intravenously as propacetamol (N, N-diethyl glycidyl ester). Propacetamol has been withdrawn from the market and intravenous paracetamol is now available. Hypersensitivity to acetaminophen seems to be rare and evidence for an IgE-mediated mechanism is anecdotal.

Plasma volume expanders (colloids)

Today, colloids have been recognized to cause up to 4% of all perioperative anaphylactic reactions. These reactions were severe in 20% of the cases and generally occurred 20 min after start of infusion. Fatalities to colloids have been reported (Freeman, 1991; Porter & Goldberg, 1986). Although the mechanisms of these reactions remain poorly understood, evidence has emerged for an IgE-mediated mechanism in some patients. It seems obvious to avoid gelatin based colloids in patients with known gelatin allergy. Diagnosis from IgE-mediated gelatin allergy is generally established upon quantification of sIgE (Phadia c74), appropriate skin tests or basophil activation assays such as histamine release tests and flow assisted quantification of *in vitro* activated basophils. In the absence of sIgE assays, diagnosis of anaphylaxis from HES generally relies upon skin tests. The clinical relevance of IgG, IgM and IgA antibodies against HES remains unknown. High-molecular-weight dextrans (40, 70 and 75 kDa) are accompanied by significant side effects including dextran-induced allergic reactions (DIAR). These are immune complex mediated by dextran-reactive antibodies of the IgG class. Severe DIAR is characterized by bronchospasm, profound hypotension, cardio-respiratory arrest and fatalities. In order to avoid this potentially life-threatening complication associated with dextran, the DIAR, hapten dextran (1kDa) is infused before starting the first application of dextran. Nevertheless, accidents still happen. Given the mechanism of DIAR, the diagnostic value of skin tests is not established. Dextran reactive antibodies can be quantified, but the technique is not readily available. Anaphylaxis from albumin is anecdotal. Egg allergy does not seem a contraindication to the administration of albumin.

Chlorhexidine and other antiseptics

Chlorhexidine salts can trigger irritant dermatitis, allergic contact dermatitis, urticaria/anaphylaxis and combined urticaria/anaphylaxis and allergic contact dermatitis. Symptoms of chlorhexidine anaphylaxis have been attributed to cutaneous, percutaneous, mucosal, and parenteral application. Life-threatening reactions with profound hypotension, ventricular fibrillation and cardiac ischaemia are generally associated with mucosal or parenteral exposure as might occur during application of urethral gels, implanted antimicrobial surgical mesh, and insertion of chlorhexidine-coated central venous catheters respectively. Severe, potentially life-threatening anaphylaxis from simple cutaneous application such as perioperative skin disinfection and wound cleansing remains anecdotal and probably underestimated. In a recent survey, chlorhexidine accounted for 27% of the overlooked perioperative hypersensitivity reactions (Garvey *et al.*, 2001). Prevalence of chlorhexidine anaphylaxis is not uniform among countries; it could be related to the concentration of chlorhexidine in antiseptics used in different countries. Up to now, diagnosis of anaphylaxis from chlorhexidine can readily established with SPT applying a 10-fold dilution of the available stock solution of chlorhexidine digluconate (2%) in alcohol (70%). In this chapter, it is also demonstrated quantification of chlorhexidine-specific IgE and flow cytometry assisted quantification of *in vitro* activated basophils to constitute reliable instruments to document anaphylaxis from chlorhexidine. The sIgE assay for chlorhexidine has now become commercially available (c8, Phadia). Although povidone-iodine (betadine) is a commonly applied topical antiseptic solution, anaphylaxis to this compound is rare. Clinical suspicion of povidone-iodine anaphylaxis was generally corroborated by skin test and basophil activation assays.

Local anaesthetics

Local anaesthetics (benzoic acid esters or amide derivatives) are commonly used during regional and general anaesthesia but their application is often not obvious and/or unmentioned in the anaesthetic reports, e.g. when applied to alleviate propofol-induced vascular pain. Although generally considered as intrinsically safer than general anaesthesia, local anaesthetics can elicit a variety of side effects. Immunological reactions to local anaesthetics, particular the newer amides, however, remain anecdotal and symptoms usually result from vasovagal episodes or anxiety reactions. Acute disorientation or seizures may occur after overdosage or inadvertent intravenous injection. In addition, many local anaesthetics contain adrenaline as a vasoconstricting agent. Local anaesthetics can also produce sympathetic effects that may include tremulousness, palpitations, tachycardia, diaphoresis, light-headedness, or near syncope, irrespective the presence or absence of vasoconstricting agents. Other excipients associated with local anaesthetics such as anti-oxidants and preservatives (bisulphites, parabens, carboxymethylcellulose, para-aminobenzoic acid) can also elicit adverse and even allergic reactions. Challenge tests remain the gold standard, or rather reference test to diagnose anaphylaxis from local anaesthetics and different protocols exist. (Soto Aguilar *et al.*, 1998).

Protamine and heparins

Protamine can cause significant histamine release resulting in (fatal) hypotension and bronchospasm, and also causes pulmonary hypertension. Previous exposure to protamine through use of protamine-containing insulins (NPH: Neutral Protamine Hagedorn) (Dykewicz *et al.*, 1994) or during heparin neutralization, vasectomy and fish allergy have been proposed to predispose to the development of untoward reactions from the subsequent use of this drug. Although skin tests with protamine may be helpful in identifying a possible IgE-mediated response in selected cases, these tests must be interpreted with caution because they do not necessarily predict clinical sensitivity and do not identify all patients at risk. A sIgE protamine is available (rc207). In rare occasions, heparins have been identified as the cause of anaesthetic anaphylaxis.

Aprotinin

Aprotinin is a naturally occurring polybasic serine protease inhibitor, purified from cattle lung. It is the only agent with class A level 1 evidence for reduction transfusion rates and return to operating theatre to control bleeding after heart surgery. Skin tests and quantification of sIgE and sIgG antibodies for aprotinin have a good negative predictive value but positive predictive value is poor.(Prieto García *et al.*, 2008).

Hyaluronidase

Hyaluronidase is a proteolytic enzyme used as an adjunct to local anaesthesia, especially in nerve blocks and ophthalmic anaesthesia. Hypersensitivity reactions towards hyaluronidase comprise local acute or delayed reactions as well as more generalized anaphylactic reactions. Diagnosis of IgE-mediated allergy to hyaluronidase can be confirmed by skin tests, quantification of sIgE or flow cytometry. (Dieleman *et al.*,2012).

Oxytocin

Oxytocin is a synthetically manufactured hormone that stimulates contractions of uterine smooth muscle and is indicated for induction and augmentation of labor as well as in abortions. Anaphylaxis from oxytocin is rare and diagnosis is generally based upon skin tests. Note that oxytocin can produce hypotension through a pharmacodynamical mechanism when given in larger intravenous boluses.

Dyes

Patent blue is an aniline dye used as antibacterial and antifungal agent, apart from its use in lymphography. Today, it is the dye of choice for intra-operative sentinel lymph node mapping for breast cancer and melanoma. Most patients have suffered from reactions during lymphography. Anaphylaxis can also result from alternative routes of administration. The second dye applied for sentinel node mapping is isosulphan blue (Lymphazurin), a derivative from patent blue. Because of the extensive cross-reactivity between isosulphan blue and patent blue, the dyes cannot be considered as reciprocal alternatives (Aydogan *et al.*, 2008). Anaphylaxis due to other blue dyes such as indigo carmine (sodium indigotin disulfonate) and methylene blue seems anecdotal. Because methylene blue has been shown to be equally effective for mapping of sentinel lymph nodes and appears not to pose an important risk for anaphylaxis, it was proposed as the dye of choice for mapping studies. Skin tests and basophil activation tests constitute confirmatory procedures for anaphylaxis from blue dyes and can contribute to the identification of potential cross-reactive and safe alternative dyes. A physical examination is required for all patients, although the extent will be guided by the history.

5   Clinical Pearls of Allergy Diagnosis

1. An accurate clinical history is the mainstay of allergy diagnosis,

2. Skin prick/serum IgE tests provide objective confirmation of IgE sensitivity,

3. Skin prick/serum IgE tests must always be interpreted in the context of the history,

4. If you do not need the result of a test then don't do the test. Indiscriminate skin prick/serum IgE panels' are more likely to confuse rather than inform diagnosis and should be avoided.

6   Conclusion

Allergy diagnosis depends primarily on the clinical history. This history, aided by a physical examination and objective tests of IgE sensitivity (either skin tests or serum IgE measurements), is used to focus on the patient's diagnosis. There should be a high index of suspicion for allergy in patients presenting with symptoms of asthma, rhinitis, or eczema, particularly if there is an associated personal or family history of other atopic disease. Whether or not allergy is suspected on the basis of the initial history, a limited number of skin prick tests or *in vitro* tests for specific IgE, including physical examination should also be performed in the majority of patients to confirm or exclude anaphylaxis.

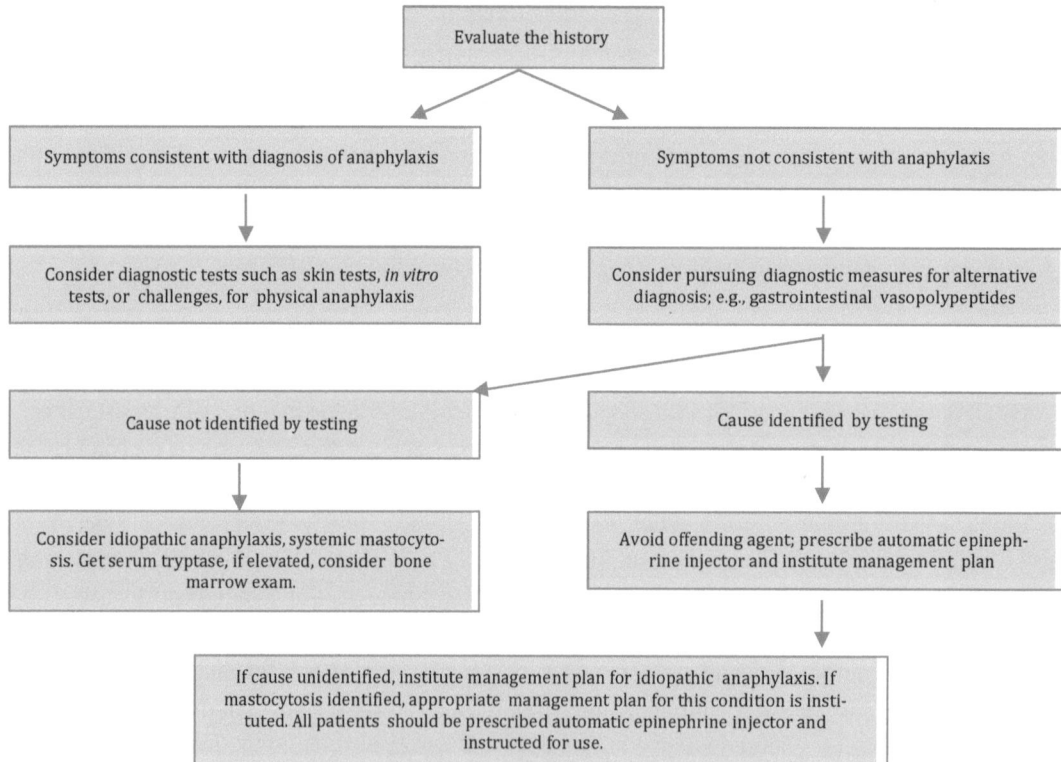

Table 3: Algorithm for diagnosis of allergic reactions

References

Cockcroft D, Davis B. (2009). *Direct and indirect challenges in the clinical assessment of asthma. Ann Allergy Asthma Immunol; 103:363–370.*

Eckman J, Saini SS, Hamilton RG. (2009). Diagnostic evaluation of food-related allergic diseases. Allergy, Asthma, and Clinical Immunology; 5:2.

Mertes PM, Laxenaire MC, Alla F. (2003). Anaphylactic and anaphylactoid reactions occurring during anesthesia in France in 1999–2000. Anesthesiology; 99: 536–545.

Caughey GH. (2006). Tryptase genetics and anaphylaxis. J Allergy Clin Immunol;117:1411–14.

Laroche D, Vergnaud MC, Sillard B, Soufarapis H, Bricard H. (1991). Biochemical markers of anaphylactoid reactions to drugs. Comparison of plasma histamine and tryptase. Anesthesiology;75: 945–949.

Schwartz LB, Irani AM, Roller K, Castells MC, Schechter NM. (1987). Quantitation of histamine, tryptase, and chymase in dispersed human T and TC mast cells. J Immunol;138: 2611–2615.

Schwartz LB, Sakai K, Bradford TR, Ren S, Zweiman B, Worobec AS et al. (1995). The alpha form of human tryptase is the predominant type present in blood at baseline in normal subjects and is elevated in those with systemic mastocytosis. J Clin Invest; 96: 2702–2710.

Edston E, Hage-Hamsten M. (1998). Beta-tryptase measurements post-mortem in anaphylactic deaths and in controls. Forensic Sci Int ;93:135–142.

Fisher MM, Baldo BA. (1998). Mast cell tryptase in anaesthetic anaphylactoid reactions. Br J Anaesth;80:26-29.

Hamilton RG. (2010). Clinical laboratory assessment of immediate-type hypersensitivity. J Allergy Clin Immunol;125:S 284–296.

Joint Task Force on Practice Parameters. (2008). Allergy diagnostic testing: an updated practice parameter. Ann Allergy Asthma Immunol; 100:S1–148.

Brockow K, Romano A, Blanca M, Ring J, Pichler W, Demoly P. (2002). General considerations for skin test procedures in the diagnosis of drug hypersensitivity. Allergy; 57:45–51.

Fisher MM, Bowey CJ. (1997). Intradermal compared with prick testing in the diagnosis of anaesthetic allergy. Br J Anaesth;79: 59–63.

Thong BY, Yeow C. (2004). Anaphylaxis during surgical and interventional procedures. Ann Allergy Asthma Immunol;92:619–628.

Fisher MM, Merefield D, Baldo B. (1999). Failure to prevent an anaphylactic reaction to a second neuromuscular blocking drug during anaesthesia. Br J Anaesth; 82:770–773.

Fisher MM, Baldo BA. (2000). Immunoassays in the diagnosis of anaphylaxis to neuromuscular blocking drugs: the value of morphine for the detection of IgE antibodies in allergic subjects. Anaesth Intensive Care;28: 167–170.

Florvaag E, Johansson SG, Oman H, Venemalm L, Degerbeck F, Dybendal T et al. (2005). Prevalence of IgE antibodies to morphine. Relation to the high and low incidences of NMBA anaphylaxis in Norway and Sweden, respectively. Acta Anaesthesiol Scand; 49: 437–444.

Gueant JL, Mata E, Monin B, Moneret-Vautrin DA, Kamel L, Nicolas JP et al. (1991). Evaluation of a new reactive solid phase for radioimmuno-assay of serum specific IgE against muscle relaxant drugs. Allergy; 46:452–458.

Abuaf N, Rajoely B, Ghazouani E, Levy DA, Pecquet C, Chabane H et al. (1999). Validation of a flow cytometric assay detecting in vitro basophil activation for the diagnosis of muscle relaxant allergy. J Allergy Clin Immunol;104(2 Pt 1):411–418.

Ebo DG, Lechkar B, Schuerwegh AJ, Bridts CH, De Clerck LS, Stevens WJ. (2002).Validation of a two-color flow cytometric assay detecting in vitro basophil activation for the diagnosis of IgE mediated natural rubber latex allergy. Allergy;57:706–712.

21.Torres MJ, Padial A, Mayorga C, Fernandez T, Sanchez-Sabate E, Cornejo-Garcia JA et al. (2004). The diagnostic interpretation of basophil activation test in immediate allergic reactions to betalactams. Clin Exp Allergy; 34:1768–1775.

Bernstein L, Li JT, Bernstein DI et al. (2008). Allergy Diagnostic Testing: An Updated Practice Parameter. Annals of Allergy, asthma, & Immunology; 100:3,S1-148

Jogie-Brahim S, Min HK, Fukuoka Y, et al. (2004). Expression of alpha tryptase and beta-tryptase by human basophils. J Allergy Clin Immunol.;113(6):1086–92.

Bhivgade S, Melkote S, Ghate S, Jerajani HR. (2012). Hereditary angioedema: not an allergy. Indian J Dermatol. ;57(6):503.

Urm SH, Yun HD, Fenta YA, Yoo KH, Abraham RS, Hagan J, Juhn YJ. (2013). Asthma and risk of selective IgA deficiency or common variable immunodeficiency: a population-based case-control study. Mayo Clin Proc.;88(8):813-21.

Singh K, Chang C, Gershwin ME. (2014). IgA deficiency and autoimmunity. Autoimmun Rev. ;13(2):163-77.

Levy JH, Gottge M, Szlam F, Zaffer R, McCall C. (2000). Wheal and flare responses to intradermal rocuronium and cisatracurium in humans. Br J Anaesth;85:844–849.

Berg CM, Heier T, Wilhelmsen V, Florvaag E. (2003). Rocuronium and cisatracurium-positive skin tests in non-allergic volunteers: determination of drug concentration thresholds using a dilution titration technique. Acta Anaesthesiol Scand;47:576–582.

Dhonneur G, Combes X, Chassard D, Merle JC. (2004). Skin sensitivity to rocuronium and vecuronium: a randomized controlled prick-testing study in healthy volunteers. Anesth Analg; 98:986–989.

Fisher M. (2004). Prick testing for neuromuscular blocking drugs. Anesth Analg; 99:1880–1881.

Tamayo E, Rodriguez-Ceron G, Gomez-Herreras JI, Fernandez A, Castrodeza J, Alvarez FJ. (2006). Prick-test evaluation to anaesthetics in patients attending a general allergy clinic. Eur J Anaesthesiol;23:1–6.

Hepner DL, Castells MC. (2003). Latex allergy: An update. Anesth Analg;96:1219 ⁻29.

Sanz ML, Garcia BE, Prieto I, Tabar A, Oehling A. (1996). Specific IgE determination in the diagnosis of beta-lactam allergy. J Investig Allergol Clin Immunol;6:89–93.

Khurana C, de Belder MA. (1999). Red-man syndrome after vancomycin: potential cross-reactivity with teicoplanin. Postgrad Med J;75:41–43.

Scherer K, Bircher AJ. (2005). Hypersensitivity reactions to fluoroquinolones. Curr Allergy Asthma Rep;5:15–21.

Marone G, Stellato C. (1992). Activation of human mast cells and basophils by general anaesthetic drugs. Monogr Allergy;30:54–73.

Karila C, Brunet-Langot D, Labbez F, Jacqmarcq O, Ponvert C, Paupe J et al. (2005). Anaphylaxis during anesthesia: results of a 12-year survey at a French pediatric center. Allergy;60:828–834.

Tomar GS, Tiwari AK, Chawla S, Mukherjee A, Ganguly S. (2012). Anaphylaxis related to fentanyl citrate. J Emerg Trauma Shock. ;5(3):257-61.

Pierzchalska M, Mastalerz L, Sanak M, Zazula M, Szczeklik A. (2000). A moderate and unspecific release of cysteinyl leukotrienes by aspirin from peripheral blood leucocytes precludes its value for aspirin sensitivity testing in asthma. Clin Exp Allergy;30:1785–1791.

Gamboa P, Sanz ML, Caballero MR, Urrutia I, Antepara I, Esparza R et al. (2004). The flow-cytometric determination of basophil activation induced by aspirin and other non-steroidal anti-inflammatory drugs (NSAIDs) is useful for in vitro diagnosis of the NSAID hypersensitivity syndrome. Clin Exp Allergy;34:1448–1457.

Gamboa PM, Sanz ML, Caballero MR, Antepara I, Urrutia I, Jauregui I et al. (2003). Use of CD63 expression as a marker of in vitro basophil activation and leukotriene determination in metamizol allergic patients. Allergy;58:312–317.

Lebel B, Messaad D, Kvedariene V, Rongier M, Bousquet J, Demoly P. (2001). Cysteinyl-leukotriene release test (CAST) in the diagnosis of immediate drug reactions. Allergy;56: 688–692.

Freeman MK. (1979) Fatal reaction to haemaccel. Anaesthesia;34: 341 ⁻3.

Porter SS, Goldberg RJ. (1986). Intraoperative allergic reaction to hydroxyl ethyl starch: A report of two cases. Can Anaesth Soc J;33:394 -8.

Garvey LH, Roed-Petersen J, Husum B. (2001). Anaphylactic reactions in anaesthetised patients: Four cases of chlorhexidine allergy. Acta Anaesthesiol Scand;45:1290 -4.

Soto -Aguilar MC, deShazo RD, Dawson ES. (1998). Approach to the patient with suspected local anesthetic sensitivity. Immunol Allergy Clin North Am;4:851 -65.

Dykewicz MS, Kim HW, Orfan N, Yoo TJ, Lieberman P. (1994). Immunologic analysis of anaphylaxis to protamine component in neutral protamine Hagedorn human insulin. J Allergy Clin Immunol; 93(1 Pt 1):117-25.

Prieto García A, Villanueva A, Lain S, Baeza ML. (2008). Fatal intraoperative anaphylaxis after aprotinin administration. J Investig Allergol Clin Immunol.;18(2):136.

Dieleman M, Bettink-Remeijer MW, Jansen J, et al. (2012). High incidence of adverse reactions to locoregional anaesthesia containing hyaluronidase after uneventful ophthalmic surgery. Acta Ophthalmol.;90(3):e245-6.

Aydogan F, Celik V, Uras C, Salihoglu Z, Topuz U. (2008). A comparison of the adverse reactions associated with isosulfan blue versus methylene blue dye in sentinel lymph node biopsy for breast cancer. Am J Surg.;195(2):277-8.

Alopecia Areata

Adel Alsantali
Department of Dermatology
King Fahd Armed Forces Hospital, Jeddah, Saudi Arabia

1   Introduction

Alopecia areata (AA) is a common nonscarring, autoimmune disease that can affect any hair-bearing area. It occurs in all ethnic groups, ages, and both sexes. The lifetime risk for AA is about 1.7% in the general population (Safavi *et al.*, 1995). Up to 60% of patients had their first AA episode before the age of 20 (Price, 1991). Although, AA is an unpredictable disease but extensive involvement and the long duration of the hair loss are the most important poor prognostic factors. Although AA is generally asymptomatic disease, it is psychologically distressing to the patients. Therapy for AA should be tailored in light of severity of the condition and patient's age. In this chapter, currently available treatments for AA are discussed, together with the clinical presentation, and pathogenesis.

2   Clinical Features

Alopecia areata most commonly presents as well demarcated round or oval totally bald patches of hair loss (Patchy AA) as shown in figure 1 and 2. Depending on the duration of the disease, patchy AA can be subclassified into AA transient (AAT; if they had a patchy hair loss for less than 1 year), AA persistent (AAP; if they had patchy hair loss for a year or more). In severe cases, the hair loss may affect all over the scalp (alopecia totalis (AT)) or the entire body hair (alopecia universalis (AU)) including the eyebrows, eyelashes, axillary and pubic hair (Figure 3).

Less common types of alopecia areata include reticular AA, ophiasis type, in which hair loss in the parietal temporo-occipital area of the scalp (figure 4) and ophiasis inversa (sisapho) which is the opposite of ophiasis type and the hair loss spares the periphery of the scalp. Alopecia areata incognita (AAI) is a type of alopecia areata characterized by acute diffuse shedding of telogen hairs without typical patches. Acute diffuse and total alopecia (ADTA) is a newly described subtype of AA that is characterized by rapid progression of diffuse alopecia and female predominance. ADTA is associated with a favorable prognosis and rapid and spontaneous recovery even without treatment (Lew *et al.*, 2009). Table1 summarizes the subtypes for AA.

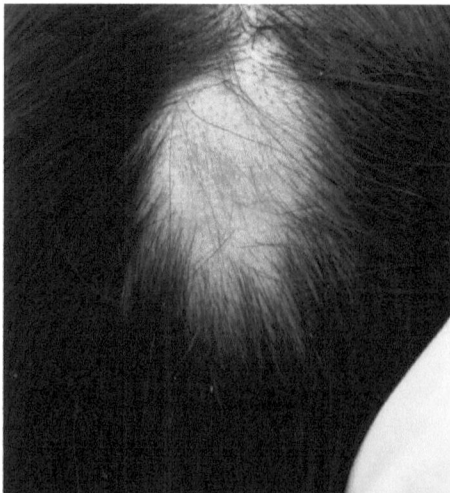

Figure 1: A solitary well demarcated patch of alopecia areata on scalp.

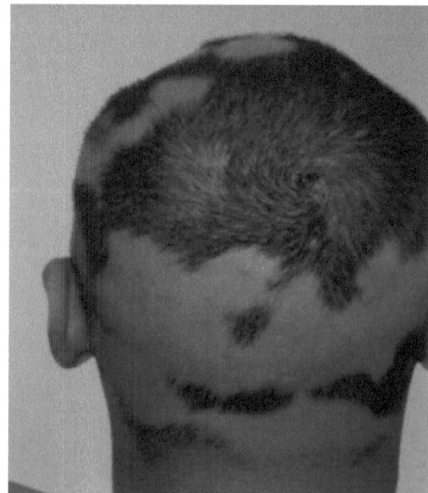

Figure 2: Multiple alopecia areata patches.

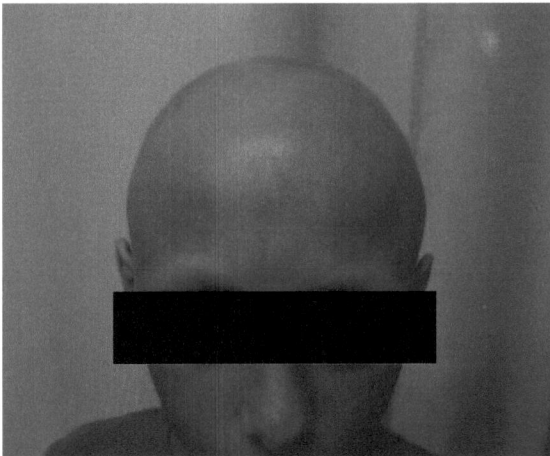

Figure 3: Alopecia universalis. Note eyebrow and eyelashes involvement.

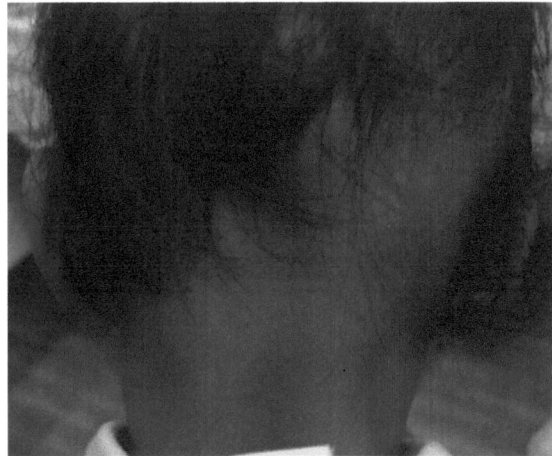

Figure 4: Ophiasis pattern of alopecia areata affecting
the periphery of the scalp.

1. According to duration of the disease:
a. AA transient (AAT): if hair loss for less than 1 year
b. AA persistent (AAP): hair loss for a year or more

2. According to the pattern of involvement
a. Patchy AA
b. Alopecia totalis (AT)
c. Alopecia universalis (AU)
d. Reticular AA
e. Ophiasis type
f. ophiasis inversa (sisapho)
g. Alopecia areata incognita (AAI)
h. Acute diffuse and total alopecia (ADTA)

Table 1: Classification of alopecia areata.

The affected skin in classic AA patches usually looks normal apart from hair loss. At the border of alopecic patches, hair pull test can be positive indicating the activity of the disease. As the hairs undergo an abrupt conversion from anagen to telogen, the affected hairs taper proximally and broken which is known as "exclamation mark hair". Although AA is usually an asymptomatic disease, it affects the patients socially and psychologically. Upon regrowth, hypopigmented white hairs usually appear first then repigmentation will follow gradually.

AA can affect the nail from 10-66% of patients. Nail pitting is the most common nail changes usually seen. Pits are usually small, superficial and regularly distributed in a geometric pattern. Other nail changes include onycholysis, koilonychia (concave nail plate) onychomadesis (shedding of the nails), brittle nails, beau's lines, red spotted lunula, trachyonychia (longitudinal ridging of the nails) and punctuate or transverse leukonychia (Madani & Shapiro, 2000).

Characteristics trichoscopic (scalp dermoscopic) features of AA include yellow dots, tapering hairs (exclamation mark hairs), broken hairs, black dots and short vellus hairs. Yellow dots are not a specific diagnostic marker for AA as they can be seen in other hair disorders like androgenetic alopecia, congenital hypotrichoses, and kerion celsi. Black dots and yellow dots correlate with disease severity whereas black dots, tapering hairs, and broken hairs correlate with disease activity (Inui *et al.*, 2008; Miteva & Tosti, 2012). The black dots can be found also in trichotillomania, which should be noted for differential diagnosis of AA. Figure 5 presents some of the trichoscopic findings that can be seen in AA.

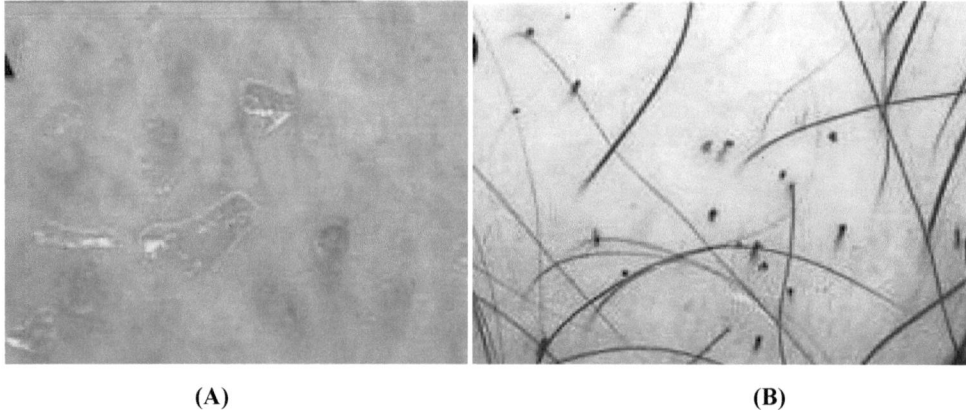

(A)   **(B)**

Figure 5: Trichoscopic features of alopecia areata: (A) yellow dots, (B) black dots (Rudnicka *et al.*, 2011).

3   Prognosis

Although AA is unpredictable disease, there are several poor prognostic indicators have been reported. The extent of the disease (AT/AU) and its chronicity are among of most important poor prognostic factors. Other prognosis signs include ophiasis pattern of hair loss, nail changes, presence of other autoimmune disease, young age at onset of the disease, and a positive family history (Madani & Shapiro, 2000). The presence of atopy has been shown to be associated with a poor prognosis (Ajith *et al.*, 2006; Ikeda, 1965; Ucak *et al.*, 2012) but some studies did not find that (van der Steen *et al.*, 1991). The rapidly progressive alopecia areata subtype, ADTA is considered to have favorable prognosis.

4   Associated Comorbidities

AA is considered as an autoimmune disease and frequently occurs in association with other autoimmune disorders such as thyroiditis (in 8% to 28%) and vitiligo (in 3% to 8% of AA patients) (Hordinsky & Ericson, 2004; Seyrafi *et al.*, 2005). In a retrospective epidemiologic study, the frequency of thyroid antibodies was significantly higher in AA patients than in control group (25.7 % vs. 3% respectively), but there was no significant association between the disease severity and the presence of these antibodies (Kasumagic-Halilovic, 2008). Autoimmune thyroiditis seems to have a higher occurrence in children with AA (up to 47.8%) (Kurtev & Iliev, 2005). So it is imperative to screen these patients for thyroid autoimmunity especially if AA is extensive and chronic.

Atopic dermatitis is 2 to 3 times more common in AA patients compared with general population (Chu *et al.*, 2011). The incidence of atopy is higher in AT/AU patients. Other reported comorbidities with

AA include Down's syndrome, autosomal recessive autoimmune polyglandular syndrome (APS-1), pernicious anemia, celiac disease, multiple sclerosis, Addison disease, ulcerative colitis, lupus erythematosus, psoriasis, and Turner's syndrome. Ocular abnormalities have been reported in AA patients. Lenticular changes in the form of punctuate opacities and cataracts were found in 40% of AA patients (Pandhi *et al.,* 2009). In another study these asymptomatic lens opacities were observed in 51% of patients (Recupero *et al.*, 1999). Also, retinal alterations were found in 41% AA subjects.

5 Differential Diagnosis

In children, AA should be differentiated from tinea capitis, trichotillomania and congenital atrichia. The alopecic patches in tinea capitis are usually associated with scaling and inflammation that may progress to severely inflame deep abscesses termed kerion. Trichotillomania is a compulsive disorder that often presents as solitary or multiple alopecic patches with broken hair of varying length that resulted from hair pulling by the patient him/herself. The other differential diagnoses that may also be considered are secondary syphilis, lupus erythematosus, telogen effluvium and traction alopecia (Table 3).

1. Autoimmune thyroid diseases
2. Vitiligo
3. Atopy (atopic dermatitis, allergic rhinitis)
4. Psychiatric morbidity (anxiety, depression and mood disturbance)
5. Ophthalmologic changes (lenticular and retinal alterations)
6. Down syndrome
7. Addison disease
8. Pernicious anemia
9. Psoriasis
10. Lupus erythematosus
11. Celiac disease
12. Ulcerative colitis
13. Multiple sclerosis
14. Autosomal recessive autoimmune polyglandular syndrome (APS-1)

Table 2: Comorbidities associated with AA

- Tinea capitis
- Trichotillomania
- Secondary syphilis
- Discoid lupus erythematosus (DLE)
- Traction alopecia
- Lichen planopilaris
- Pseudopelade of Brocq
- Alopecia mucinosa
- Congenital atrichia
- Telogen effluvium

Table 3: AA differential diagnosis

6   Investigation

In most cases, the diagnosis of AA is straightforward and based on the clinical presentation. Skin biopsy and fungal cultures may be considered in difficult cases. Routine screening tests for the associated auto-immune diseases is not generally recommended. But as stated before it is wise to screen for autoimmune thyroid disease particularly in chronic extensive AA (AT/AU).

7   Histopathology

Depending on the disease duration, four stages can be defined in the histopathology of AA: acute, sub-acute, chronic, and recovery. The classic histopathologic finding of AA is the perifollicular and intrafol-licular lymphocytic (CD4+, CD8+) infiltrate which is described as appearing similar to a swarm of bees (Figure 6). This characteristic feature occurs in the acute phase of AA but may be absent in a late stages of the disease (Dy & Whiting, 2011). The lymphocytic infiltrate in AA is usually deep in subcutis sparing the bulge area where the stem cell is located. Other histopathologic findings in the acute phase include apoptosis, necrosis, edema and foreign body granulomatous reactions. Pigment incontinence can also be seen which is due to melanocytes destruction in the apex of dermal papillae. The presence of eosinophils has been reported to be a useful feature in the diagnosis of difficult cases (Peckham *et al.*, 2011). In a sub-acute phase, there is a significant decrease in the anagen: telogen and catagen ratio. Also the vellus hairs increase whereas the terminal hairs decrease. The lymphocytic and eosinophilic infiltrates may be seen in the follicular streamers (nonsclerotic fibrous tracts that extend along the original site of the previ-ous terminal hair follicles into the subcutis.) Follicular miniaturization and the presence of nanogen folli-cles (an intermediate stage between terminal and vellus hairs) are usually evident in the chronic stage of the disease (Figure 7). The terminal to vellus (T:V) hair ratio declines to 1.3:1 (normal T:V ratio is 7:1). In the recovery stage, there is little or no inflammation. As the miniaturized hairs grow, the terminal hairs increases and T:V ratio returns to normal (Whiting, 2003).

8   Pathogenesis

Although the pathogenesis of AA is not fully understood, T-lymphocyte mediated inflammatory changes, autoimmunity, neuropeptides, genetics and pyschologic distress have been reported to be factors in the development of AA.

8.1   Autoimmunity

AA is a T-lymphocyte mediated autoimmune disease. The presence of peribulbar inflammatory infil-trates, the association of AA with other autoimmune disease and the hair regrowth with immunosuppres-sive therapies are great evidences for the autoimmune pathogenesis. In a normal hair follicle, keratino-cytes does not express major histocompatibility complex (MHC) class I and II antigens and there are only a few Langerhans cells around and within hair follicles. Also, several immunosuppressive cytokines are expressed prominently by the follicular epithelium. These findings suggest that the hair follicle is an im-mune privileged site. However, in AA this immune privilege seem to be lost as there are an increased expression of MHC-I and II, and a decrease of the immunosuppressive molecules (Gilhar, 2010).

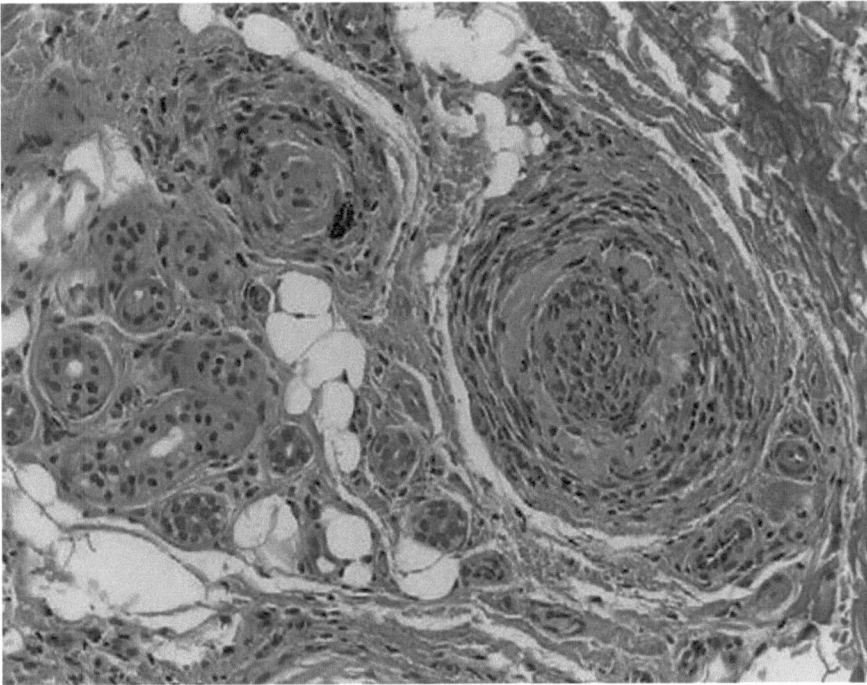

Figure 6: Acute alopecia areata. Horizontal section: classic peribulbar lymphocytic infiltrate (Hematoxylin-eosin stain; original magnification:×20).

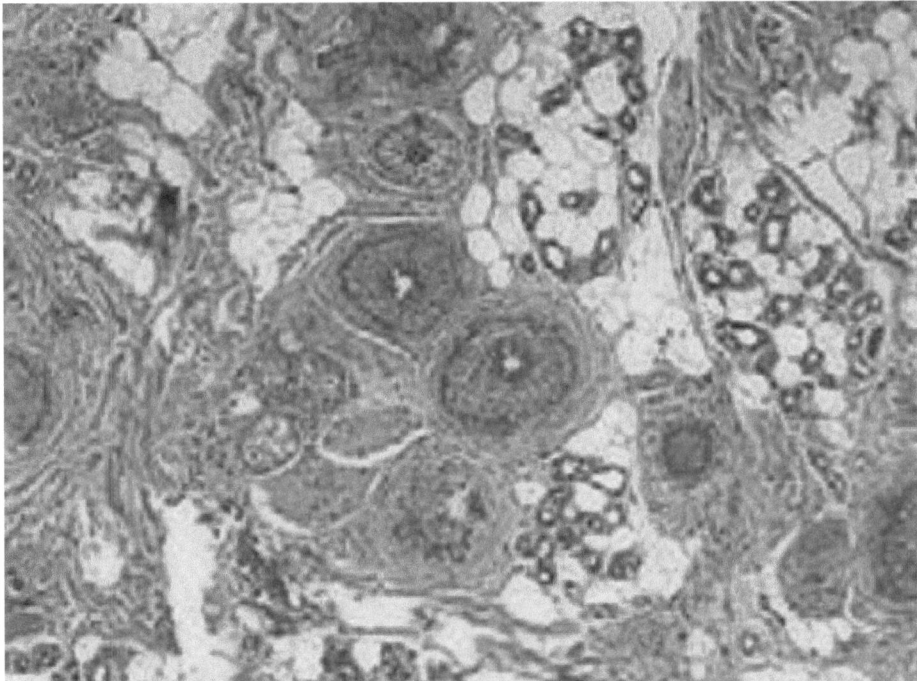

Figure 7: Chronic alopecia areata. Horizontal section: marked miniaturization and on inflammation. (Hematoxylin-eosin stain; original magnification:×4).

Moreover, the expression of adhesion molecules (ICAM-2 and ELAM-1) have been shown to be increased in the peribulbar and perivascular areas of AA affected skin. These changes lead to targeting the hair follicles by the inflammatory cells and the development of AA. Activated cytotoxic T-lymphocytes produce tumor necrosis factors, Fas ligands, and granzymes which lead to hair follicle apoptosis (Kalkan *et al.*, 2013). CD8+ T-lymphocytes seem to have a primary role in hair follicle damage whereas CD4+ cells have a helper role in the process (McElwee *et al.*, 2005). Why the immune privilege for the hair follicle is lost in AA patients and what are the initial events leading to the development of AA? The cause or causes for the collapse of immune privilege are not clear but, it has been suggested that events such as stress, infection, or microtrauma might lead to downregulation of the immunosuppressive cytokines. The onset of AA may be due to abnormal regression of catagen hair leading to hair follicle antigen uptake and presentation to lymphocytes (Botchkareva *et al.*, 2006). From mice studies, proinflammatory changes started in skin draining lymph nodes several weeks before the onset of alopecia or even before lymphocytic infiltration of the skin (Zoller *et al.*, 2002).

Recently oxidative stress has come to light as a possible triggering factor for autoimmune diseases. In a case-control study, the mean serum total oxidant capacity, malondialdehyde, and the oxidative stress index were found to be significantly higher in AA patients than in the control group and correlate with disease severity (Bakry *et al.*, 2013). Other studies showed an increase in lipid peroxidation and defective antioxidant activity of superoxide dismutase in patients with AA (Abdel Fattah *et al.*, 2011; Koca *et al.*, 2005). Whether these changes play a role in disease pathogenesis or result from the inflammatory process needs further investigation. Also, the role of antioxidants in AA treatment and prevention warrant further clinical studies.

8.1.1   Humoral Immunity

Hair follicle specific IgG antibody has been shown to be increased in the blood of AA patients. However, the injections of these autoantibodies in different models did not prove a significant role of these autoantibodies in the development of AA. Of notes, antithyroid and anti nuclear antibodies can be found more in AA patients than in normal population (Grandolfo *et al.*, 2008; Yano *et al.*, 1999).

8.2   Genetics

AA is considered an autoimmune disease with genetic background due to the following:

1. High frequency of a family history of AA in affected people particularly in patients with early onset AA (range from 10% to 42%).

2. Concordance rate in identical twins was repeated up to 55%.

3. Although the lifetime risk for AA is about 1.7% in the general population, the estimated lifetime risk of the disease is 7.1% in siblings, 7.8% in parents, and 5.7% in offsprings of AA patients. The first genome-wide association study (GWAS) identified at least eight regions in the genome (Petukhova *et al.*, 2010). These eight regions implicated genes of the immune system, as well as genes that are unique to the hair follicle itself.

(i) Chromosome 2q33.2 containing the CTLA4 gene;

(ii) Chromosome 4q27 containing the IL2/IL21 locus;

(iii) Chromosome 6p21.32 containing the HLA class II region;

(iv) Chromosome 6q25.1 which harbors the cytomegalovirus UL16-binding protein (ULBP) gene cluster;

(v) Chromosome 9q31.1 containing syntaxin 17 (STX17);

(vi) Chromosome 10p15.1 containing IL-2 receptor A (IL-2RA; CD25;

(vii) Chromosome 11q13 containing peroxiredoxin 5 (PRDX5);

(viii) Chromosome 12q13 containing Eos (also known as Ikaros family zinc finger 4; IKZF4).

These genomic region contain several genes that control the activation and proliferation of regulatory T cells, cytotoxic T-lymphocyte – associated antigen 4 (CTL4), interleukin (IL)-2/IL-21, IL-2 receptor A (IL-2RA; CD25) and Eos, as well as the human leukocyte antigen (HLA) region. A region of strong association was found within ULBP (cytomegalovirus UL16 binding protein) gene cluster in chromosome 6q25.1. ULBP3 and ULBP6 genes make the natural killer cell receptor NKG2D activating ligands or signal that can trigger the NKG2D receptor initiating an autoimmune response. NKG2DLs are stress-induced molecules that act as "danger signals" to alert NK and CD8T lymphocytes through the engagement of the activating receptor, NKG2D. AA hair follicle dermal sheath showed a greater expression of ULBP3. Another two GWASs confirm these findings and add new susceptibility loci for AA. These loci are for IL-13, KIAA0350/CLEC16A and SPATA5 (spermatogenesis-associated protein 5) gene on chromosome 4 (Forstbauer *et al.*, 2012; Jagielska *et al.*, 2012). The GWASs implicated both innate and adaptive immunity in the pathogenesis of AA. These findings suggest new approaches of exploration for therapy based on the underlying mechanisms of AA with a focus not only on T cells, but on cells that express the NKG2D receptor as well.

8.3 Stress

Psychosocial stress has been reported to play a role in the onset and the progression of alopecia areata but controlled clinical studies were not conclusive. Some studies showed a positive relationship between the stress and AA (Manolache & Benea, 2007; Taheri *et al.*, 2012). In the other hand, some did not find a significant relation between AA and stressful events (Brajac *et al.*, 2003). Some studies have shown that AA patients have a higher reactivity to stress and higher scores for depression than normal population (Chu *et al.*, 2012). Experimental studies in mice with alopecia areata showed a marked increase in the hypothalamic-pituitary-adrenal (HPA) axis tone and activity centrally, and peripherally in the skin and lymph nodes. Stress further exacerbated changes in AA mouse HPA activity. The positive correlation of HPA hormone levels with skin Th1 cytokines suggests that altered HPA activity may occur as a consequence of the immune response associated with AA (Zhang *et al.*, 2009).

AA itself can cause a severe psychological distress, depression and anxiety. Also, there is a high psychiatric comorbidity (up to 78%) in AA (mainly as generalized anxiety disorder, depression, and mood disorders) requiring systematic psychiatric evaluation and treatments. In alopecia areata, like in some other diseases, psychosomatics and immunology are not opposed because immune cells are controlled by the nervous system through neurotransmitters. Stress may increase the production of neuropeptides such as substance P (SP) which induces accumulation of CD8+ cells and induce these cells to produce large amounts of IFN-γ. Also, SP may stimulate the production of nerve growth factor, which in turn induces mast cells accumulation and degranulation around hair follicles leading to hair follicle regression.

8.4   The effect of AA on hair follicle growth cycle

Normal hair follicles pass through 3 phases: the growth phase (anagen), the regression phase (catagen), and the resting phase (telogen). Several possible pathologic patterns of hair cycle can be seen in AA which include, dystrophic anagen in which the hair follicle are unable to produce hair fibers, truncated cycling (hairs cycle through multiple anagen – telogen phases of brief duration) and prolonged telogen phase without attempt to produce hair follicle (in chronic AA) (Freyschmidt-Paul *et al.*, 2008). The severity of inflammation and the chronicity of the disease may play a role in determining the nature and the pattern of the hair cycle derangement (Whiting, 2003). More than one hair cycle pattern can occur in the same AA patient.

9   Treatment

Many therapeutic modalities have been used to treat alopecia areata, with variable efficacy and safety profiles. Unfortunately, none of these agents is curative or preventive. Also, many of these therapeutic agents have not been subjected to randomized, controlled trials, and, except for topical immunotherapy, there are few published studies on long-term outcomes. In the view of the author, the therapeutic agents are organized according to their efficacy and safety profiles into first-line, second-line, and third-line options. Usually, there is a lag time from initiation of therapy to hair regrowth. This lag time varies from one therapeutic agent to another and it is usually about 3-6 months. This lag time should be kept in mind, so as not abandon therapy before having allowed a minimum time for response. Of note, the lag time is shorter with intralesional and systemic corticosteroids than other agents (Chartaux & Joly, 2010).

9.1   First-line therapies

9.1.1   Intralesional corticosteroids

Several studies have shown the efficacy of intralesional corticosteroid injections. Abell and Munro reported hair regrowth in 71% of patients with subtotal alopecia areata treated by triamcinolone acetonide injections and in 7% of a placebo group (Abell & Munro, 1973). For limited scalp alopecia areata, intralesional corticosteroid therapy is considered as the drug of choice by many experts. The most widely used agent is triamcinolone acetonide. Different concentrations of triamcinolone acetonide are used, in the range of 2.5–10 mg/ml, but 5 mg/ml is the preferred concentration for the scalp and face. A maximum volume of 3 ml on the scalp in one visit is recommended. Corticosteroid is injected into the deep dermis level or just beneath the dermis in the upper subcutis. The injections can be repeated at 4–6 weekly intervals. The use of mesotherapy multi-injectors with 5–7 needles is an alternative approach to decrease injection pain and to make the procedure more homogenous. Side effects include skin atrophy and telangiectasia which can be minimized by the use of smaller volumes and avoiding superficial injections. To alleviate injection pain, topical anesthetic may be applied 30–60 minutes before the treatment. Although the effect of a single intralesional corticosteroid injection has been observed to persist for up to 9 months, reported relapse rates were 29% in limited alopecia areata and 72% in alopecia totalis during a 3-month follow-up period. Patients who received intralesional triamcinolone acetonide therapy for long time (cumulative dose greater than 500 mg) should be screened for osteoporosis and monitored for effects on bone mineral density (Samrao *et al.*, 2013).

9.1.2   Topical corticosteroids

Many forms of topical corticosteroids have been prescribed for alopecia areata, including creams, gels, ointments, lotions, and foams. Sixty-one percent of patients using 0.1% betamethasone valerate foam achieved more than 75% hair regrowth in comparison with 27% in the 0.05% betamethasone dipropionate lotion group (Mancuso *et al.*, 2003). Topical corticosteroids are far less effective in alopecia totalis and alopecia universalis. A highly potent topical corticosteroid under occlusion is the preferred method when using topical corticosteroids. Folliculitis is a common side effect to topical corticosteroids. Telangiectasia and atrophy may develop rarely. The reported relapse rate is 37%–63% (Tosti *et al.*, 2003).

9.1.3   Minoxidil

In a placebo-controlled, double-blind study, hair regrowth was observed in 63.6% and 35.7% of the minoxidil-treated and placebo groups, respectively (Price, 1987a). However, only 27% of the minoxidil-treated patients showed cosmetically acceptable hair regrowth. In another study, hair regrowth was achieved in 38% and 81% of patients treated with 1% and 5% topical minoxidil, respectively (Fiedler-Weiss, 1987). Most studies have shown no beneficial effect of topical minoxidil in alopecia totalis and alopecia universalis (Price, 1987b). Minoxidil 5% solution or foam is frequently used with other therapeutic agents as an adjuvant therapy. The adverse effects of topical minoxidil include contact dermatitis and facial hypertrichosis.

9.1.4   Anthralin

A few controlled trials have assessed the efficacy of topical anthralin in the treatment of alopecia areata. In an open study, a cosmetic response was seen in 25% of patients with severe alopecia areata treated using 0.5%–1.0% anthralin cream (Fiedler-Weiss & Buys, 1987). In another trial, combination therapy of 5% minoxidil and 0.5% anthralin was used to treat 51 patients with severe alopecia areata; only 11% of patients achieved cosmetically acceptable hair regrowth (Fiedler *et al.*, 1990). Anthralin needs to be applied in a high enough concentration (0.5%–1%) and sufficiently frequently (daily) to produce a mild irritant reaction in order to be effective. Severe irritation and staining of skin and clothes are some of the possible adverse events with anthralin.

9.1.5   Topical immunotherapy

Topical sensitizers that have been used in the treatment of alopecia areata include diphenylcyclopropenone (DPCP), squaric acid dibutylester (SADBE), and dinitrochlorobenzene. Dinitrochlorobenzene is no longer used because it was shown to be mutagenic in the Ames test (Strobel & Rohrborn, 1980). DPCP is the topical sensitizer of choice. SADBE is expensive and not stable in ace-tone. DPCP is light sensitive and should be protected from light. Initially the patient is sensitized using a 2% solution of DPCP applied to a 4×4 cm area of the scalp. After two weeks, 0.001% DPCP solution is applied to the same half of the scalp. The DPCP concentration is increased gradually every week until mild dermatitis is observed (Orecchia & Perfetti, 1991). The solution should be on the scalp for 48 hours. The scalp should be protected from the sun during this time. Once hair regrowth is obtained on the treated half of the scalp, both sides are treated. Both sides of the scalp can be treated from the start also. DPCP is applied on a weekly basis by a trained nurse. If there is no response after 6 months of treatment, DPCP can be discontinued. SADBE may be tried in poor responders to DPCP or in those who do not develop a sensitization to 2% DPCP. SADBE is applied once or twice per week. The adverse effects to topical sensitizers include cervical lymphadenopathy, a severe eczematous reaction, urticaria, and postinflammatory pigment changes. The response rate of alopecia totalis/alopecia universalis patients to DPCP was 17.4% in the largest reported diphenylcyclopropenone study, whereas the cumulative patient response was 77% (Wiseman *et al.*, 2001). Several negative prognostic factors in the treatment of alopecia areata with DPCP have been suggested, including long duration of disease, alopecia totalis/alopecia universalis, nail changes, atopy, and family history of alopecia areata. Recurrence of alopecia areata after achieving significant hair regrowth developed in 62.6% of patients. In a retrospective study of 121 patients with extensive alopecia areata, fexofenadine hydrochloride has been shown to enhance the efficacy of topical immunotherapy (Inui *et al.*, 2009). The mechanism of action of topical sensitizers could be due to perifollicular lymphocyte apoptosis, changes in the peribulbar CD4/CD8 lymphocyte ratio, and antigenic competition (Wasylyszyn *et al.*, 2007).

9.1.6   Prostaglandin analogs

Eyelash hypertrichosis is a common adverse effect to the use of these antiglaucoma eye drops (Hart & Shafranov, 2004). Some case series did not show an effect in the treatment of eyelashes in patients with alopecia areata (Roseborough *et al.*, 2009). In a nonrandomized, controlled study of latanoprost (a prostaglandin F2 α analog) eye drops in patients with alopecia universalis, acceptable results (total and moderate hair regrowth) were achieved in 45% of patients (Coronel-Perez *et al.*, 2010). In another retrospective trial, 0.03% bimatoprost eye drops were used once a day for one year. Complete regrowth of the eyelashes was noted in 24.3% of patients and moderate growth in 18.9% of treated subjects (Vila *et al.*, 2010). Relapses were observed in 17.5% of the patients, mainly in the slight response group.

9.1.7   Topical retinoids

In a comparative study of topical tretinoin 0.05%, topical betamethasone dipropionate lotion, and dithranol paste 0.25%, a good response has been seen in 55% of patients treated with topical tretinoin in comparison with 70% and 35% in the topical steroid and dithranol groups, respectively (Das *et al.*, 2010). Although the mechanism for its action in alopecia areata is not completely understood, the associated tretinoin-induced dermatitis might contribute to regrowth in alopecia areata. Larger, double-blind, placebo-controlled trials are needed.

9.1.8   Bexarotene

In a randomized bilateral half-head study, hair regrowth of at least 50% on treated sites was noticed in only 26% of patients treated with 1% bexarotene gel (Talpur *et al.*, 2009). Mild irritation is a common side effect.

9.1.9   Capsaicin

In a nonblinded randomized study, 9.5% of patients with alopecia areata showed cosmetically acceptable hair regrowth after 12 weeks of applying capsaicin ointment (Ehsani *et al.*, 2009).

9.2 Second-line therapies

9.2.1 Sulfasalazine

Sulfasalazine is a combination of sulfapyridine and 5-aminosalicylic acid linked by a diazo bond. Sulfasalazine has both immunomodulatory and immunosuppressive actions that include suppression of T cell proliferation and reducing the synthesis of cytokines, including interleukin (IL) 6, 1, and 12, tumor necrosis factor alpha, and antibody production (Ranganath & Furst, 2007). Sulfasalazine has been used safely as a long-term treatment of various inflammatory and autoimmune diseases, including inflammatory bowel disease and rheumatoid arthritis. Several case reports and case series showed good hair regrowth with sulfasalazine in the treatment of alopecia areata. In an uncontrolled prospective trial of sulfasalazine in 39 patients with persistent alopecia areata, hair regrowth of more than 60% was achieved in 25.6% of patients. A moderate response was seen in 30.7% of patients (Rashidi & Mahd, 2008). Also, in another uncontrolled open-label study, complete hair regrowth was reported in 27.3% of subjects (Aghaei, 2008). Sulfasalazine was started at 500 mg twice daily for one month, 1 g twice daily for one month, and then 1 g three times daily (Ellis *et al.*, 2002). Side effects to sulfasalazine include gastrointestinal distress, dizziness, and headache. Gastrointestinal symptoms can be minimized by using enteric-coated tablets, taking the medication with food, and starting at lower doses. Initially, patients should have a complete blood count, liver function tests, creatinine, and glucose-6-phosphate dehydrogenase level measurement. Complete blood counts and liver function tests should be performed at 2–4-week intervals during the first three months of therapy. The reported relapse rates are 22.7%–45.5%.

9.2.2   Photochemotherapy

The success rate for oral and topical psoralen plus ultraviolet A (PUVA) ranged from 15% to more than 70% (Mohamed *et al.*, 2005; Taylor & Hawk, 1995). PUVA turban is a method of administering a dilute psoralen solution (8-methoxypsoralen 0.0001%) selectively to the scalp for 20 minutes using a cotton towel as a turban. The patient's scalp is then exposed to ultraviolet A radiation. Treatment sessions are performed two or three times per week. PUVA- turban has been shown to be effective in about 70% of treated patients (Behrens-Williams *et al.*, 2001; Broniarczyk-Dyla *et al.*, 2006). During a follow-up period of 15 months after PUVA-turban therapy, recurrences of alopecia areata were observed in 26% of responders. PUVA-turban therapy lacks the systemic side effects of oral PUVA and can be considered as alternative therapy for patients with alopecia areata.

9.2.3   Excimer laser

In a treatment of 42 alopecia areata patches with the 308 nm excimer laser, hair regrowth was observed in 41.5% of treated areas (Al-Mutairi, 2007). Hair regrowth was noticed to begin to appear during the second month of therapy. No regrowth of hair was noted on the control patches. Laser therapy was administered twice a week for a maximum of 24 sessions. Apart from erythema at the treated sites, there were no significant adverse effects. Relapses of alopecia areata were observed in two patients with patchy alopecia areata of the scalp who had shown complete regrowth earlier. Also, the use of excimer laser in children with alopecia areata has been reported to have a good success rate (Al-Mutairi, 2009).

9.2.4   Fractional photothermolysis laser

Good hair regrowth was achieved with fractional Er: Glass laser in a single case report (Yoo *et al.*, 2010). Randomized controlled trials in a larger number of patients are required to confirm the efficacy of this modality of treatment.

9.3   Third-line therapies

9.3.1   Systemic corticosteroids

Systemic corticosteroids are one of the commonly prescribed therapies in patients with extensive alopecia areata. Various forms of corticosteroids have been used in different regimens. In one study, a once-monthly oral pulse of 300 mg prednisone induced a complete response in 41% of patients (Ait Ourhroui et al., 2010). A similar effect has been reported in a placebo-controlled trial of oral prednisolone 200 mg once weekly in the treatment of extensive alopecia areata (Kar et al., 2005). The relapse rate was 25%, and side effects of the therapy were noted in 55% of patients. In a comparative trial, the response rate was better in patients treated with intramuscular triamcinolone acetonide 40 mg once monthly than in those treated with oral dexamethasone 0.5 mg/day (Kurosawa et al., 2006). In the same study, impairment of adrenocortical reserve was seen in 23% of the intramuscular triamcinolone acetonide group and in 7% of patients treated with oral prednisolone pulse therapy of 80 mg for 3 consecutive days once every 3 months. In a study of 139 patients treated with pulse corticosteroid therapy, a good response was achieved in 59.4% of patients with recent-onset disease (duration of alopecia areata up to 6 months) in comparison with 15.8% of subjects who had had alopecia areata for more than 6 months (Nakajima et al., 2007). Alopecia totalis and alopecia universalis are far less responsive to this therapy than patchy alopecia areata (Friedli et al., 1998). The use of systemic corticosteroids is limited by their side effects (hyperglycemia, weight gain, hypertension, adrenal suppression, dysmenorrhea, immunosuppression, and acneiform eruption) (Lester et al., 1998) and the high relapse rate (14%–100%).

9.3.2   Methotrexate

In a long-term follow-up study of methotrexate in 33 patients with alopecia areata, complete hair regrowth was achieved in 57% and 63% of patients who used methotrexate alone or with low doses of oral corticosteroids (prednisone 10–20 mg/day), respectively (Chartaux & Joly, 2010). Thirty percent of patients had partial hair regrowth. The weekly dosages of methotrexate were 15–25 mg. The onset of hair regrowth was seen after a median delay of three months. Recurrences of alopecia areata after a decrease of the methotrexate dose or after stopping treatment were observed in 57% (8/14 cases) of responders. In a retrospective trial of methotrexate in 14 children with alopecia areata, approximately one third of patients experienced a clinically relevant therapeutic response (Royer et al., 2011). The mean age of the patients was 14.7 (range 8–18) years. Adverse effects to methotrexate include persistent nausea, transient elevation of hepatic enzymes, and leucopenia.

9.3.3   Cyclosporine

The success rate with oral cyclosporine is 25%–76.6% (Kim et al., 2008; Shapiro et al., 1997). A recent study showed that a good response to oral cyclosporine can be predicted if the serum level of IL-18 is elevated and the level of soluble IL-2 receptor is low (Lee et al., 2010). The use of oral cyclosporine in patients with alopecia areata is not generally favored due to its adverse event profile (nephrotoxicity, immune suppression, and hypertension) and a high relapse rate (up to 100%).(Gupta et al., 1990). Also, alopecia areata incidence has been reported in several organ transplant patients receiving cyclosporine (Cerottini et al., 1999; Phillips et al., 2005). Although hypertrichosis is a documented side effect of oral cyclosporine, a good response has not been achieved by using topical cyclosporine in humans (Gilhar et al., 1989).

9.3.4   Azathioprine

Azathioprine, a thiopurine analog immunosuppressive drug, has been used to treat a vast array of auto-immune diseases. It inhibits DNA synthesis and thus decreases proliferation of cells, especially T and B lymphocytes. Azathioprine also decreases the number of Langerhans cells and other antigen-presenting cells in the skin. In a recent pilot study of 20 patients treated with azathioprine 2 mg/kg/day as monotherapy, mean hair regrowth was 52.3% (Farshi et al., 2010). These results need to be confirmed in large-scale, randomized, controlled studies.

9.3.5   Biologics

Although tumor necrosis factor alpha is implicated in the pathogenesis of alopecia areata, there are several reported cases that have shown either development of alopecia areata or complete failure to respond to different tumor necrosis factor alpha inhibitors, including adalimumab (Garcia Bartels et al., 2006; Kirshen & Kanigsberg, 2009), infliximab (Ettefagh et al., 2004; Fabre & Dereure, 2008), and etanercept (Pan & Rao, 2009; Posten & Swan, 2005). In a prospective trial of 17 patients with alopecia areata, Strober et al. concluded that etanercept does not effectively treat moderate to severe alopecia areata (Strober et al., 2005). Also, in a placebo-controlled study, Price et al showed that efalizumab, an anti-CD11a antibody, is not effective in the treatment of alopecia areata (Price et al., 2008). Some clinical trials are ongoing to evaluate the efficacy of the newer biologic therapies in the treatment of alopecia areata.

9.4   Psychological support

Alopecia areata is considered to be an example of a psychosomatic disorder, leading to dramatic and devastating emotions which can negatively impact patient self-esteem, body image, and self-confidence (Ruiz-Doblado, Carrizosa, & Garcia-Hernandez, 2003). One important step that should not be overlooked during the course of management of alopecia areata is offering psychological support to foster increased self-esteem and adaptation to this disease. Helping patients with alopecia areata cope with depression and an unpredictable disease like alopecia areata can be achieved by several ways, including education of the patient about the nature of disease, psychotherapy, hypnotherapy, antidepressants, and support groups (Abedini, Farshi, Mirabzadeh, & Keshavarz, 2013). Hypnotherapy may significantly improve depression, anxiety, and quality of life, but not hair regrowth (Willemsen, Haentjens, Roseeuw, & Vanderlinden, 2010). Patients with extensive disease may wear scalp prostheses, such as wigs, hairpieces, or other scalp coverings.

9.5   Other therapies

Other therapeutic agents have been tried, with some degree of success. These modalities include aromatherapy (Hay et al., 1998), a combination of topical garlic gel and betamethasone valerate cream (Hajheydari et al., 2007), topical azelic acid (Sasmaz & Arican, 2005), oral zinc supplementation (Bhat et al., 2009; H. Park et al.,2009), topical onion juice (Sharquie & Al-Obaidi, 2002), a simvastatin-ezetimibe combination (Ali & Martin, 2010; Robins, 2007), inosiplex (Georgala et al., 2006), and intralesional injections of candida antigen (Rosenberg & Skinner, 2006). These treatment modalities need to be confirmed in large scale, double-blind, placebo-controlled trials. There are other modalities of therapy that have not shown good efficacy. These agents include imiquimod (D'Ovidio et al., 2002; Koc et al., 2008), topical calcineurin inhibitors (S. W. Park et al., 2002; Price et al., 2005; Rigopoulos et al., 2007), botulinum toxin type A (Cho *et al.*, 2010), topical tri-iodothyronine ointment (Nasiri *et al.*, 2012), photo-dynamic therapy (Yoo *et al.*, 2010), and topical 5-Fluorouracil (Kaplan & Olsen, 2004).

9.6   Management plan

Treatment options should be selected according to patient age and extent of disease. For patients younger than 10 years, a combination of 5% minoxidil solution twice daily with mid-potent topical corticosteroids should be tried first. If there is no good improvement after 6 months, short-contact anthralin is considered as second-line therapy. Excimer laser can be used, particularly in patchy alopecia areata.

For patients older than 10 years of age with alopecia areata involving less than 50% of the scalp, intralesional triamcinolone acetonide injection (5 mg/cc) is the recommended option for treatment. If there is no good response after 6 months, other options can be tried, including potent topical corticosteroids under occlusion at night, 5% topical minoxidil twice a day, short-contact anthralin, and excimer laser.

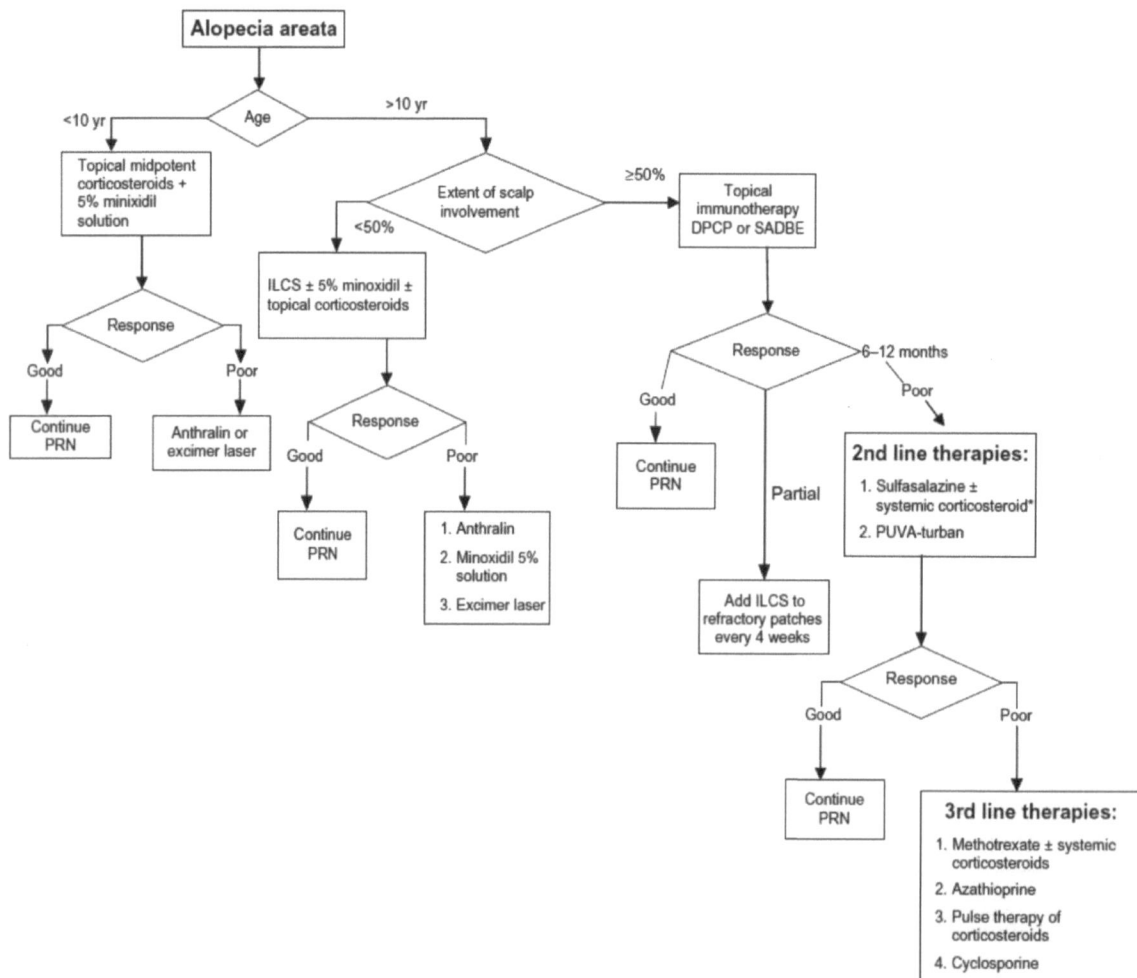

Figure 8: Treatment plan for alopecia areata. DPCP, diphenylcyclopropenone; ILCS, intralesional corticosteroids; PRN, as needed; SADBE, squaric acid dibutylester. *Systemic Corticosteroids are used as a bridge therapy.

If alopecia areata involves more than 50% of the scalp, topical immunotherapy with DPCP is the first therapeutic option recommended by many experts in hair diseases. Intralesional injections of triamcinolone acetonide are used to treat persistent alopecic patches.

For patients who respond poorly to DPCP and those who cannot use it, second-line therapies can be used. Several review articles of alopecia areata therapy suggest topical minoxidil and topical corticosteroids (Alkhalifah *et al.*, 2010; Madani & Shapiro, 2000; Ross & Shapiro, 2005; Wasserman *et al.*, 2007) but, as discussed earlier, the yield of these topical agents in the treatment of extensive alopecia areata is limited. Therefore, we suggest that patients with extensive resistant disease can use sulfasalazine with or without systemic corticosteroids. Systemic steroids are used as bridge therapy until the sulfasalazine takes effect. Treatment with sulfasalazine is generally well tolerated and characterized by a lower incidence of serious side effects in comparison with other systemic therapies like corticosteroids and methotrexate. The other second-line therapy is PUVA turban. It is a well tolerated therapy with minimal local phototoxic side effects and without the systemic side effects of PUVA. These options are selected based on a balance between the efficacy and safety of these therapeutic agents.

If these therapies fail or are not tolerated, third-line therapeutic options can be discussed with patients in terms of the expected outcome of therapy and possible side effects. These agents include methotrexate with or without a systemic corticosteroid, azathioprine, cyclosporine, and pulse therapy of corticosteroids. While using these drugs, close monitoring of patients is important to avoid possible side effects. A summary of an alopecia areata treatment plan is shown as an algorithmic approach in Figure 8.

References

Abdel Fattah, N. S., Ebrahim, A. A., & El Okda, E. S. (2011). Lipid peroxidation/antioxidant activity in patients with alopecia areata. *J Eur Acad Dermatol Venereol, 25(4)*, 403-408.

Abedini, H., Farshi, S., Mirabzadeh, A., & Keshavarz, S. (2013). Antidepressant effects of citalopram on treatment of alopecia areata in patients with major depressive disorder. *J Dermatolog Treat*.

Abell, E., & Munro, D. D. (1973). Intralesional treatment of alopecia areata with triamcinolone acetonide by jet injector. *Br J Dermatol, 88(1)*, 55-59.

Aghaei, S. (2008). An uncontrolled, open label study of sulfasalazine in severe alopecia areata. *Indian J Dermatol Venereol Leprol, 74(6)*, 611-613.

Ait Ourhroui, M., Hassam, B., & Khoudri, I. (2010). [Treatment of alopecia areata with prednisone in a once-monthly oral pulse]. *Ann Dermatol Venereol, 137(8-9)*, 514-518.

Ajith, C., Gupta, S., & Kanwar, A. J. (2006). Efficacy and safety of the topical sensitizer squaric acid dibutyl ester in Alopecia areata and factors influencing the outcome. *J Drugs Dermatol, 5(3)*, 262-266.

Al-Mutairi, N. (2007). 308-nm excimer laser for the treatment of alopecia areata. *Dermatol Surg, 33(12)*, 1483-1487.

Al-Mutairi, N. (2009). 308-nm excimer laser for the treatment of alopecia areata in children. *Pediatr Dermatol, 26(5)*, 547-550.

Ali, A., & Martin, J. M. t. (2010). Hair growth in patients alopecia areata totalis after treatment with simvastatin and ezetimibe. *J Drugs Dermatol, 9(1)*, 62-64.

Alkhalifah, A., Alsantali, A., Wang, E., McElwee, K. J., & Shapiro, J. (2010). Alopecia areata update: part II. Treatment. *J Am Acad Dermatol, 62(2)*, 191-202, quiz 203-194.

Bakry, O. A., Elshazly, R. M., Shoeib, M. A., & Gooda, A. (2013). Oxidative Stress in Alopecia Areata: A Case-Control Study. *Am J Clin Dermatol*.

Behrens-Williams, S. C., Leiter, U., Schiener, R., Weidmann, M., Peter, R. U., & Kerscher, M. (2001). The PUVA-turban as a new option of applying a dilute psoralen solution selectively to the scalp of patients with alopecia areata. J Am Acad Dermatol, 44(2), 248-252.

Bhat, Y. J., Manzoor, S., Khan, A. R., & Qayoom, S. (2009). Trace element levels in alopecia areata. Indian J Dermatol Venereol Leprol, 75(1), 29-31.

Botchkareva, N. V., Ahluwalia, G., & Shander, D. (2006). Apoptosis in the hair follicle. J Invest Dermatol, 126(2), 258-264.

Brajac, I., Tkalcic, M., Dragojevic, D. M., & Gruber, F. (2003). Roles of stress, stress perception and trait-anxiety in the onset and course of alopecia areata. J Dermatol, 30(12), 871-878.

Broniarczyk-Dyla, G., Wawrzycka-Kaflik, A., Dubla-Berner, M., & Prusinska-Bratos, M. (2006). Effects of psoralen-UV-A-Turban in alopecia areata. Skinmed, 5(2), 64-68.

Cerottini, J. P., Panizzon, R. G., & de Viragh, P. A. (1999). Multifocal alopecia areata during systemic cyclosporine A therapy. Dermatology, 198(4), 415-417.

Chartaux, E., & Joly, P. (2010). [Long-term follow-up of the efficacy of methotrexate alone or in combination with low doses of oral corticosteroids in the treatment of alopecia areata totalis or universalis]. Ann Dermatol Venereol, 137(8-9), 507-513.

Cho, H. R., Lew, B. L., Lew, H., & Sim, W. Y. (2010). Treatment effects of intradermal botulinum toxin type A injection on alopecia areata. Dermatol Surg, 36 Suppl 4, 2175-2181.

Chu, S. Y., Chen, Y. J., Tseng, W. C., Lin, M. W., Chen, T. J., Hwang, C. Y., et al. (2011). Comorbidity profiles among patients with alopecia areata: the importance of onset age, a nationwide population-based study. J Am Acad Dermatol, 65(5), 949-956.

Chu, S. Y., Chen, Y. J., Tseng, W. C., Lin, M. W., Chen, T. J., Hwang, C. Y., et al. (2012). Psychiatric comorbidities in patients with alopecia areata in Taiwan: a case-control study. Br J Dermatol, 166(3), 525-531.

Coronel-Perez, I. M., Rodriguez-Rey, E. M., & Camacho-Martinez, F. M. (2010). Latanoprost in the treatment of eyelash alopecia in alopecia areata universalis. J Eur Acad Dermatol Venereol, 24(4), 481-485.

D'Ovidio, R., Claudatus, J., & Di Prima, T. (2002). Ineffectiveness of imiquimod therapy for Alopecia Totalis/Universalis. J Eur Acad Dermatol Venereol, 16(4), 416-417.

Das, S., Ghorami, R. C., Chatterjee, T., & Banerjee, G. (2010). Comparative assessment of topical steroids, topical tretenoin (0.05%) and dithranol paste in alopecia areata. Indian J Dermatol, 55(2), 148-149.

Dy, L. C., & Whiting, D. A. (2011). Histopathology of alopecia areata, acute and chronic: Why is it important to the clinician? Dermatol Ther, 24(3), 369-374.

Ehsani, A. H., Toosi, S., Seirafi, H., Akhyani, M., Hosseini, M., Azadi, R., et al. (2009). Capsaicin vs. clobetasol for the treatment of localized alopecia areata. J Eur Acad Dermatol Venereol, 23(12), 1451-1453.

Ellis, C. N., Brown, M. F., & Voorhees, J. J. (2002). Sulfasalazine for alopecia areata. J Am Acad Dermatol, 46(4), 541-544.

Ettefagh, L., Nedorost, S., & Mirmirani, P. (2004). Alopecia areata in a patient using infliximab: new insights into the role of tumor necrosis factor on human hair follicles. Arch Dermatol, 140(8), 1012.

Fabre, C., & Dereure, O. (2008). Worsening alopecia areata and de novo occurrence of multiple halo nevi in a patient receiving infliximab. Dermatology, 216(2), 185-186.

Farshi, S., Mansouri, P., Safar, F., & Khiabanloo, S. R. (2010). Could azathioprine be considered as a therapeutic alternative in the treatment of alopecia areata? A pilot study. Int J Dermatol, 49(10), 1188-1193.

Fiedler-Weiss, V. C. (1987). Topical minoxidil solution (1% and 5%) in the treatment of alopecia areata. J Am Acad Dermatol, 16(3 Pt 2), 745-748.

Fiedler-Weiss, V. C., & Buys, C. M. (1987). Evaluation of anthralin in the treatment of alopecia areata. Arch Dermatol, 123(11), 1491-1493.

Fiedler, V. C., Wendrow, A., Szpunar, G. J., Metzler, C., & DeVillez, R. L. (1990). Treatment-resistant alopecia areata. Response to combination therapy with minoxidil plus anthralin. Arch Dermatol, 126(6), 756-759.

Forstbauer, L. M., Brockschmidt, F. F., Moskvina, V., Herold, C., Redler, S., Herzog, A., et al. (2012). Genome-wide pooling approach identifies SPATA5 as a new susceptibility locus for alopecia areata. Eur J Hum Genet, 20(3), 326-332.

Freyschmidt-Paul P, McElwee KJ, Hoffmann R. (2008). Alopecia areata. In: Whiting DA, Blume-Peytavi U, Tosti A, editors. Hair growth and disorders. Berlin: Springer; pp. 311-332.

Friedli, A., Labarthe, M. P., Engelhardt, E., Feldmann, R., Salomon, D., & Saurat, J. H. (1998). Pulse methylprednisolone therapy for severe alopecia areata: an open prospective study of 45 patients. J Am Acad Dermatol, 39(4 Pt 1), 597-602.

Garcia Bartels, N., Lee, H. H., Worm, M., Burmester, G. R., Sterry, W., & Blume-Peytavi, U. (2006). Development of alopecia areata universalis in a patient receiving adalimumab. Arch Dermatol, 142(12), 1654-1655.

Georgala, S., Katoulis, A. C., Befon, A., Georgala, K., & Stavropoulos, P. G. (2006). Inosiplex for treatment of alopecia areata: a randomized placebo-controlled study. Acta Derm Venereol, 86(5), 422-424.

Gilhar, A. (2010). Collapse of immune privilege in alopecia areata: coincidental or substantial? J Invest Dermatol, 130(11), 2535-2537.

Gilhar, A., Pillar, T., & Etzioni, A. (1989). Topical cyclosporin A in alopecia areata. Acta Derm Venereol, 69(3), 252-253.

Grandolfo, M., Biscazzi, A. M., & Pipoli, M. (2008). Alopecia areata and autoimmunity. G Ital Dermatol Venereol, 143(5), 277-281.

Gupta, A. K., Ellis, C. N., Cooper, K. D., Nickoloff, B. J., Ho, V. C., Chan, L. S., et al. (1990). Oral cyclosporine for the treatment of alopecia areata. A clinical and immunohistochemical analysis. J Am Acad Dermatol, 22(2 Pt 1), 242-250.

Hajheydari, Z., Jamshidi, M., Akbari, J., & Mohammadpour, R. (2007). Combination of topical garlic gel and betamethasone valerate cream in the treatment of localized alopecia areata: a double-blind randomized controlled study. Indian J Dermatol Venereol Leprol, 73(1), 29-32.

Hart, J., & Shafranov, G. (2004). Hypertrichosis of vellus hairs of the malar region after unilateral treatment with bimatoprost. Am J Ophthalmol, 137(4), 756-757.

Hay, I. C., Jamieson, M., & Ormerod, A. D. (1998). Randomized trial of aromatherapy. Successful treatment for alopecia areata. Arch Dermatol, 134(11), 1349-1352.

Hordinsky, M., & Ericson, M. (2004). Autoimmunity: alopecia areata. J Investig Dermatol Symp Proc, 9(1), 73-78.

Ikeda, T. (1965). A new classification of alopecia areata. Dermatologica, 131(6), 421-445.

Inui, S., Nakajima, T., Nakagawa, K., & Itami, S. (2008). Clinical significance of dermoscopy in alopecia areata: analysis of 300 cases. Int J Dermatol, 47(7), 688-693.

Inui, S., Nakajima, T., Toda, N., & Itami, S. (2009). Fexofenadine hydrochloride enhances the efficacy of contact immunotherapy for extensive alopecia areata: Retrospective analysis of 121 cases. J Dermatol, 36(6), 323-327.

Jagielska, D., Redler, S., Brockschmidt, F. F., Herold, C., Pasternack, S. M., Garcia Bartels, N., et al. (2012). Follow-up study of the first genome-wide association scan in alopecia areata: IL13 and KIAA0350 as susceptibility loci supported with genome-wide significance. J Invest Dermatol, 132(9), 2192-2197.

Kalkan, G., Ates, O., Karakus, N., & Sezer, S. (2013). Functional polymorphisms in cell death pathway genes FAS and FAS ligand and risk of alopecia areata. Arch Dermatol Res.

Kaplan, A. L., & Olsen, E. A. (2004). Topical 5-fluorouracil is ineffective in the treatment of extensive alopecia areata. J Am Acad Dermatol, 50(6), 941-943.

Kar, B. R., Handa, S., Dogra, S., & Kumar, B. (2005). Placebo-controlled oral pulse prednisolone therapy in alopecia areata. J Am Acad Dermatol, 52(2), 287-290.

Kasumagic-Halilovic, E. (2008). Thyroid autoimmunity in patients with alopecia areata. Acta Dermatovenerol Croat, 16(3), 123-125.

Kim, B. J., Min, S. U., Park, K. Y., Choi, J. W., Park, S. W., Youn, S. W., et al. (2008). Combination therapy of cyclosporine and methylprednisolone on severe alopecia areata. J Dermatolog Treat, 19(4), 216-220.

Kirshen, C., & Kanigsberg, N. (2009). Alopecia areata following adalimumab. J Cutan Med Surg, 13(1), 48-50.

Koc, E., Tunca, M., Akar, A., & Kurumlu, Z. (2008). Lack of efficacy of topical imiquimod in the treatment of patchy alopecia areata. Int J Dermatol, 47(10), 1088-1089.

Koca, R., Armutcu, F., Altinyazar, C., & Gurel, A. (2005). Evaluation of lipid peroxidation, oxidant/antioxidant status, and serum nitric oxide levels in alopecia areata. Med Sci Monit, 11(6), CR296-299.

Kurosawa, M., Nakagawa, S., Mizuashi, M., Sasaki, Y., Kawamura, M., Saito, M., et al. (2006). A comparison of the efficacy, relapse rate and side effects among three modalities of systemic corticosteroid therapy for alopecia areata. Dermatology, 212(4), 361-365.

Kurtev, A., & Iliev, E. (2005). Thyroid autoimmunity in children and adolescents with alopecia areata. Int J Dermatol, 44(6), 457-461.

Lee, D., Hong, S. K., Park, S. W., Hur, D. Y., Shon, J. H., Shin, J. G., et al. (2010). Serum levels of IL-18 and sIL-2R in patients with alopecia areata receiving combined therapy with oral cyclosporine and steroids. Exp Dermatol, 19(2), 145-147.

Lester, R. S., Knowles, S. R., & Shear, N. H. (1998). The risks of systemic corticosteroid use. Dermatol Clin, 16(2), 277-288.

Lew, B. L., Shin, M. K., & Sim, W. Y. (2009). Acute diffuse and total alopecia: A new subtype of alopecia areata with a favorable prognosis. J Am Acad Dermatol, 60(1), 85-93.

Madani, S., & Shapiro, J. (2000). Alopecia areata update. J Am Acad Dermatol, 42(4), 549-566; quiz 567-570.

Mancuso, G., Balducci, A., Casadio, C., Farina, P., Staffa, M., Valenti, L., et al. (2003). Efficacy of betamethasone valerate foam formulation in comparison with betamethasone dipropionate lotion in the treatment of mild-to-moderate alopecia areata: a multicenter, prospective, randomized, controlled, investigator-blinded trial. Int J Dermatol, 42(7), 572-575.

Manolache, L., & Benea, V. (2007). Stress in patients with alopecia areata and vitiligo. J Eur Acad Dermatol Venereol, 21(7), 921-928.

McElwee, K. J., Freyschmidt-Paul, P., Hoffmann, R., Kissling, S., Hummel, S., Vitacolonna, M., et al. (2005). Transfer of CD8(+) cells induces localized hair loss whereas CD4(+)/CD25(-) cells promote systemic alopecia areata and CD4(+)/CD25(+) cells blockade disease onset in the C3H/HeJ mouse model. J Invest Dermatol, 124(5), 947-957.

Miteva, M., & Tosti, A. (2012). Hair and scalp dermatoscopy. J Am Acad Dermatol, 67(5), 1040-1048.

Mohamed, Z., Bhouri, A., Jallouli, A., Fazaa, B., Kamoun, M. R., & Mokhtar, I. (2005). Alopecia areata treatment with a phototoxic dose of UVA and topical 8-methoxypsoralen. J Eur Acad Dermatol Venereol, 19(5), 552-555.

Nakajima, T., Inui, S., & Itami, S. (2007). Pulse corticosteroid therapy for alopecia areata: study of 139 patients. Dermatology, 215(4), 320-324.

Nasiri, S., Haghpanah, V., Taheri, E., Heshmat, R., Larijani, B., & Saeedi, M. (2012). Hair regrowth with topical triiodothyronine ointment in patients with alopecia areata: a double-blind, randomized pilot clinical trial of efficacy. J Eur Acad Dermatol Venereol, 26(5), 654-656.

Orecchia, G., & Perfetti, L. (1991). Alopecia areata and topical sensitizers: allergic response is necessary but irritation is not. Br J Dermatol, 124(5), 509.

Pan, Y., & Rao, N. A. (2009). Alopecia areata during etanercept therapy. Ocul Immunol Inflamm, 17(2), 127-129.

Pandhi, D., Singal, A., Gupta, R., & Das, G. (2009). Ocular alterations in patients of alopecia areata. J Dermatol, 36(5), 262-268.

Park, H., Kim, C. W., Kim, S. S., & Park, C. W. (2009). The therapeutic effect and the changed serum zinc level after zinc supplementation in alopecia areata patients who had a low serum zinc level. Ann Dermatol, 21(2), 142-146.

Park, S. W., Kim, J. W., & Wang, H. Y. (2002). Topical tacrolimus (FK506): treatment failure in four cases of alopecia universalis. Acta Derm Venereol, 82(5), 387-388.

Peckham, S. J., Sloan, S. B., & Elston, D. M. (2011). Histologic features of alopecia areata other than peribulbar lymphocytic infiltrates. J Am Acad Dermatol, 65(3), 615-620.

Petukhova, L., Duvic, M., Hordinsky, M., Norris, D., Price, V., Shimomura, Y., et al. (2010). Genome-wide association study in alopecia areata implicates both innate and adaptive immunity. Nature, 466(7302), 113-117.

Phillips, M. A., Graves, J. E., & Nunley, J. R. (2005). Alopecia areata presenting in 2 kidney-pancreas transplant recipients taking cyclosporine. J Am Acad Dermatol, 53(5 Suppl 1), S252-255.

Posten, W., & Swan, J. (2005). Recurrence of alopecia areata in a patient receiving etanercept injections. Arch Dermatol, 141(6), 759-760.

Price, V. H. (1987a). Double-blind, placebo-controlled evaluation of topical minoxidil in extensive alopecia areata. J Am Acad Dermatol, 16(3 Pt 2), 730-736.

Price, V. H. (1987b). Topical minoxidil (3%) in extensive alopecia areata, including long-term efficacy. J Am Acad Dermatol, 16(3 Pt 2), 737-744.

Price, V. H. (1991). Alopecia areata: clinical aspects. J Invest Dermatol, 96(5), 68S.

Price, V. H., Hordinsky, M. K., Olsen, E. A., Roberts, J. L., Siegfried, E. C., Rafal, E. S., et al. (2008). Subcutaneous efalizumab is not effective in the treatment of alopecia areata. J Am Acad Dermatol, 58(3), 395-402.

Price, V. H., Willey, A., & Chen, B. K. (2005). Topical tacrolimus in alopecia areata. J Am Acad Dermatol, 52(1), 138-139.

Ranganath, V. K., & Furst, D. E. (2007). Disease-modifying antirheumatic drug use in the elderly rheumatoid arthritis patient. Rheum Dis Clin North Am, 33(1), 197-217.

Rashidi, T., & Mahd, A. A. (2008). Treatment of persistent alopecia areata with sulfasalazine. Int J Dermatol, 47(8), 850-852.

Recupero, S. M., Abdolrahimzadeh, S., De Dominicis, M., Mollo, R., Carboni, I., Rota, L., et al. (1999). Ocular alterations in alopecia areata. Eye (Lond), 13 (Pt 5), 643-646.

Rigopoulos, D., Gregoriou, S., Korfitis, C., Gintzou, C., Vergou, T., Katrinaki, A., et al. (2007). Lack of response of alopecia areata to pimecrolimus cream. Clin Exp Dermatol, 32(4), 456-457.

Robins, D. N. (2007). Case reports: alopecia universalis: hair growth following initiation of simvastatin and ezetimibe ther-apy. J Drugs Dermatol, 6(9), 946-947.

Roseborough, I., Lee, H., Chwalek, J., Stamper, R. L., & Price, V. H. (2009). Lack of efficacy of topical latanoprost and bimatoprost ophthalmic solutions in promoting eyelash growth in patients with alopecia areata. J Am Acad Dermatol, 60(4), 705-706.

Rosenberg, E. W., & Skinner, R. B., Jr. (2006). Immunotherapy of alopecia areata with intralesional Candida antigen. Pediatr Dermatol, 23(3), 299.

Ross, E. K., & Shapiro, J. (2005). Management of hair loss. Dermatol Clin, 23(2), 227-243.

Royer, M., Bodemer, C., Vabres, P., Pajot, C., Barbarot, S., Paul, C., et al. (2011). Efficacy and tolerability of methotrexate in severe childhood alopecia areata. Br J Dermatol, 165(2), 407-410.

Rudnicka, L., Olszewska, M., Rakowska, A., & Slowinska, M. (2011). Trichoscopy update 2011. J Dermatol Case Rep, 5(4), 82-88.

Ruiz-Doblado, S., Carrizosa, A., & Garcia-Hernandez, M. J. (2003). Alopecia areata: psychiatric comorbidity and adjustment to illness. Int J Dermatol, 42(6), 434-437.

Safavi, K. H., Muller, S. A., Suman, V. J., Moshell, A. N., & Melton, L. J., 3rd. (1995). Incidence of alopecia areata in Olmsted County, Minnesota, 1975 through 1989. Mayo Clin Proc, 70(7), 628-633.

Samrao, A., Fu, J. M., Harris, S. T., & Price, V. H. (2013). Bone mineral density in patients with alopecia areata treated with long-term intralesional corticosteroids. J Drugs Dermatol, 12(2), e36-40.

Sasmaz, S., & Arican, O. (2005). Comparison of azelaic acid and anthralin for the therapy of patchy alopecia areata: a pilot study. Am J Clin Dermatol, 6(6), 403-406.

Seyrafi, H., Akhiani, M., Abbasi, H., Mirpour, S., & Gholamrezanezhad, A. (2005). Evaluation of the profile of alopecia areata and the prevalence of thyroid function test abnormalities and serum autoantibodies in Iranian patients. BMC Dermatol, 5, 11.

Shapiro, J., Lui, H., Tron, V., & Ho, V. (1997). Systemic cyclosporine and low-dose prednisone in the treatment of chronic severe alopecia areata: a clinical and immunopathologic evaluation. J Am Acad Dermatol, 36(1), 114-117.

Sharquie, K. E., & Al-Obaidi, H. K. (2002). Onion juice (Allium cepa L.), a new topical treatment for alopecia areata. J Dermatol, 29(6), 343-346.

Strobel, R., & Rohrborn, G. (1980). Mutagenic and cell transforming activities of 1-chlor-2,4-dinitrobenzene (DNCB) and squaric-acid-dibutylester (SADBE). Arch Toxicol, 45(4), 307-314.

Strober, B. E., Siu, K., Alexis, A. F., Kim, G., Washenik, K., Sinha, A., et al. (2005). Etanercept does not effectively treat moderate to severe alopecia areata: an open-label study. J Am Acad Dermatol, 52(6), 1082-1084.

Taheri, R., Behnam, B., Tousi, J. A., Azizzade, M., & Sheikhvatan, M. R. (2012). Triggering role of stressful life events in patients with alopecia areata. Acta Dermatovenerol Croat, 20(4), 246-250.

Talpur, R., Vu, J., Bassett, R., Stevens, V., & Duvic, M. (2009). Phase I/II randomized bilateral half-head comparison of topical bexarotene 1% gel for alopecia areata. J Am Acad Dermatol, 61(4), 592 e591-599.

Taylor, C. R., & Hawk, J. L. (1995). PUVA treatment of alopecia areata partialis, totalis and universalis: audit of 10 years' experience at St John's Institute of Dermatology. Br J Dermatol, 133(6), 914-918.

Tosti, A., Piraccini, B. M., Pazzaglia, M., & Vincenzi, C. (2003). Clobetasol propionate 0.05% under occlusion in the treatment of alopecia totalis/universalis. J Am Acad Dermatol, 49(1), 96-98.

Ucak, H., Cicek, D., Demir, B., Erden, I., & Ozturk, S. (2012). Prognostic factors that affect the response to topical treatment in patchy alopecia areata. J Eur Acad Dermatol Venereol.

van der Steen, P. H., van Baar, H. M., Happle, R., Boezeman, J. B., & Perret, C. M. (1991). Prognostic factors in the treatment of alopecia areata with diphenylcyclopropenone. J Am Acad Dermatol, 24(2 Pt 1), 227-230.

Vila, O. T., & Camacho Martinez, F. M. (2010). Bimatoprost in the treatment of eyelash universalis alopecia areata. Int J Trichology, 2 (2), 86-88.

Wasserman, D., Guzman-Sanchez, D. A., Scott, K., & McMichael, A. (2007). Alopecia areata. Int J Dermatol, 46(2), 121-131.

Wasylyszyn, T., Kozlowski, W., & Zabielski, S. L. (2007). Changes in distribution pattern of CD8 lymphocytes in the scalp in alopecia areata during treatment with diphencyprone. Arch Dermatol Res, 299(5-6), 231-237.

Whiting, D. A. (2003). Histopathologic features of alopecia areata: a new look. Arch Dermatol, 139(12), 1555-1559.

Willemsen, R., Haentjens, P., Roseeuw, D., & Vanderlinden, J. (2010). Hypnosis in refractory alopecia areata significantly improves depression, anxiety, and life quality but not hair regrowth. J Am Acad Dermatol, 62(3), 517-518.

Wiseman, M. C., Shapiro, J., MacDonald, N., & Lui, H. (2001). Predictive model for immunotherapy of alopecia areata with diphencyprone. *Arch Dermatol, 137(8), 1063-1068.*

Yano, S., Ihn, H., Nakamura, K., Okochi, H., & Tamaki, K. (1999). *Antinuclear and antithyroid antibodies in 68 Japanese patients with alopecia areata. Dermatology, 199(2), 191.*

Yoo, K. H., Kim, M. N., Kim, B. J., & Kim, C. W. (2010). *Treatment of alopecia areata with fractional photothermolysis laser. Int J Dermatol, 49(7), 845-847.*

Yoo, K. H., Lee, J. W., Li, K., Kim, B. J., & Kim, M. N. (2010). *Photodynamic therapy with methyl 5-aminolevulinate acid might be ineffective in recalcitrant alopecia totalis regardless of using a microneedle roller to increase skin penetration. Dermatol Surg, 36(5), 618-622.*

Zhang, X., Yu, M., Yu, W., Weinberg, J., Shapiro, J., & McElwee, K. J. (2009). *Development of alopecia areata is associated with higher central and peripheral hypothalamic-pituitary-adrenal tone in the skin graft induced C3H/HeJ mouse model. J Invest Dermatol, 129(6), 1527-1538.*

Zoller, M., McElwee, K. J., Engel, P., & Hoffmann, R. (2002). *Transient CD44 variant isoform expression and reduction in CD4(+)/CD25(+) regulatory T cells in C3H/HeJ mice with alopecia areata. J Invest Dermatol, 118(6), 983-992.*

Mycolactone: A Target for Treatment of Buruli Ulcer

Alvar Grönberg
Molecular Dermatology, Department of Medicine
Center for Molecular Medicine, Karolinska Institutet, Sweden

Malin Jägestedt
Unit Infectious Diseases, Department of Medicine
Karolinska Institutet, Sweden

Sven Britton
Unit Infectious Diseases, Department of Medicine
Karolinska Institutet, Sweden

1   Introduction

An outbreak of an ulcerating disease, Bairnsdale ulcer, in Australia 1948 led to the identification of a mycobacterium, *M. ulcerans* (MU) as the causative agent (MacCallum *et al.*, 1948). A later large outbreak of the same disease in the Buruli region in Uganda 1960 resulted in the now more commonly used name of the disease, Buruli ulcer (Clancey *et al.*, 1961). This infectious disease has been described in 33 countries, but is mostly found in rural West Africa, Central Africa, New Guinea, Latin America and tropical regions of Asia (http://www.who.int/buruli/en/). Sporadic cases are still reported in Australia.

Buruli ulcer (BU) is considered to be a non-contagious disease. The route of infection is still unclear, but several observations suggest infections are transmitted via water-living insects (Marsollier *et al.*, 2002). The infected site, often on a lower extremity or an arm, develops into a nodule, which later progresses into a painless necrotic cutaneous lesion. Some patients develop lesions in bone or joints, either as a result of lesions that directly penetrate the skin or from hematogenous spread of bacteria. A large area around the original ulceration may rapidly be affected and can cover up to 15% of the body surface. Successful treatment of the infection usually leads to healing of the ulcer, but if the affected area is large and covers joints, scar formation is often leading to disabling contractures. Clinical observations from Buruli ulcer (BU) patients in West Africa suggest that severe MU infections can cause skeletal muscle atrophy leading to significant impairment of function (Stienstra *et al.*, 2005).

No single antibiotic has as yet proven clinically effective in combating MU infection and BU. Animal studies have shown that certain combinations of antibiotics like rifampicin and amikacin or streptomycin are effective against infection (Dega *et al.*, 2000; Dega *et al.*, 2002). A small clinical trial in Ghana confirmed that treatment with rifampin and streptomycin for 4 weeks or more inhibited growth of MU in human tissue (Etuaful *et al.*, 2005). This led to the currently recommended antibiotic regimen, which is a combination of rifampicin and streptomycin/amikacin for eight weeks as a first-line treatment for all forms of the active disease[1]. Nodules or uncomplicated cases can be treated without hospitalization. Before 2004, surgery and skin transplants were the only available treatments of BU. Surgery is still used mainly to remove necrotic tissue, cover skin defects and rectify deformities.

Daily intramuscular injections of streptomycin require hospitalization or frequent hospital visits. New treatment regimens in development are therefore attempting to find effective combinations of oral drugs. A randomized open-labeled trial using four weeks of intramuscular streptomycin and oral rifampicin followed by 4 weeks of oral rifampicin and clarithromycin had similar efficacy to 8 weeks of intramuscular streptomycin and oral rifampicin (Nienhuis *et al.*, 2010), and a pilot study of oral treatment with rifampicin and clarithromycin on 30 patients demonstrated healing in all patients (Chauty *et al.*, 2011).

Published studies of antibiotic treatment demonstrate a cure rate of >95% with a low recurrence of ulcer (≤1%) within a period of 1 year, if combined with surgery in non-healing patients (Kibadi *et al.*, 2010; Nienhuis *et al.*, 2010; Sarfo *et al.*, 2010). As many as 30% of subjects may experience what is termed a paradoxical reaction, in which the patients experience a transient lesion increase peaking around the end of the antibiotic treatment (Nienhuis *et al.*, 2010). This is believed to be due to an increased immune response to bacterial antigens (O'Brien *et al.*, 2009) as the bacterial load diminishes during therapy. This is akin to an "immune reconstitution syndrome" in HIV (Lipman & Breen 2006) or to a reversal reaction in leprosy (Wade 1955), although the latter can appear before, during or after treatment cessation.

---

[1] (WHO. Geneva: 2004. Provisional guidance on the role of specific antibiotics in the management of *Mycobacterium ulcerans* disease [Buruli ulcer]. www.who.int/buruli/information/antibiotics/en/)

MU is multiplying slowly with an initial intracellular growth phase in macrophages and a subsequent extracellular spread and growth of the bacteria. The explanation behind the extracellular spread and rapid ulceration is the MU specific toxin mycolactone (ML). This substance is released by the bacteria, spreads in tissue and blood and affects many cell types in a manner that acts in favor of bacterial survival in the host. This chapter will describe properties of ML and highlight recent discoveries concerning this molecule that may open up avenues for new treatments with more effective healing of BU.

2   Mycolactone

The cardinal feature of BU, a necrotic focus with bacterial colonization from which necrosis is spreading, suggested that MU produced a soluble cytotoxic mediator (Connor & Lunn 1966). This mediator was present in sterile filtrates of MU (George *et al.*, 1998), and ML was subsequently isolated and characterized (George *et al.*, 1999). In vitro experiments confirmed ML´s cytopathic effect, and it caused BU-like lesions when inoculated intradermally in guinea-pigs (George *et al.*, 1999; George *et al.*, 2000).

Several subsequent studies have confirmed the pivotal role of ML in ulceration. Most importantly, an ML negative strain of MU fails to cause lesions in a guinea-pig infection model (Adusumilli *et al.*, 2005). Considering ML´s essential role in BU pathogenesis, it stands out as an attractive target in the control of BU.

ML is believed to be responsible for the extracellular localization of bacteria and modulation of immunological responses to MU (Adusumilli *et al.*, 2005). Observations in experimentally infected rodents suggested that high toxin concentrations rapidly kill inflammatory cells by necrosis. At lower toxin concentrations more distant from the necrotic center, inflammatory cells die via apoptosis resulting in release of extracellular bacteria, which become surrounded by an area of coagulation necrosis. In contrast, self-healing granulomatous lesions develop after infection with a ML-negative mutant (Oliveira *et al.*, 2005).

3   Properties of Mycolactone

3.1   Chemical

ML is a polyketide-derived 12-membered ring macrolide with a highly unsaturated polyketide side-chain attached via an ester linkage (George *et al.*, 1999). Several isoforms differing in the degree of side chain methylation have been isolated from clinical specimens (Mve-Obiang *et al.*, 2003), isoform A/B being associated with potent cytopathic effects.

A cluster of genes located on a plasmid in MU encodes polyketide synthases and polyketide-modifying enzymes responsible for synthesis of ML (Stinear et al., 2004).

ML is a secreted heat-stable molecule (George *et al.*, 2000). However, ML is sensitive to light exposure as demonstrated by us (Figure 1), and others (Marion *et al.*, 2012; Xing *et al.*, 2012). In initial experiments, we showed that exposure to ultraviolet (UV) light (UV-A) at a dose (10 J/cm^2), corresponding to 30 minutes of sunlight, abolished the cytotoxic activity of ML (unpublished results). Even a 15 min exposure of ML in a water solution to sunlight via a window caused a substantial reduction of cytotoxic activity (Figure 1). Marion et al. (Marion *et al.*, 2012) demonstrated by quantitative analysis that 30 min exposure to sunlight reduced by 50% ML in acetonitrile or acetone solution contained in a glass tube. At

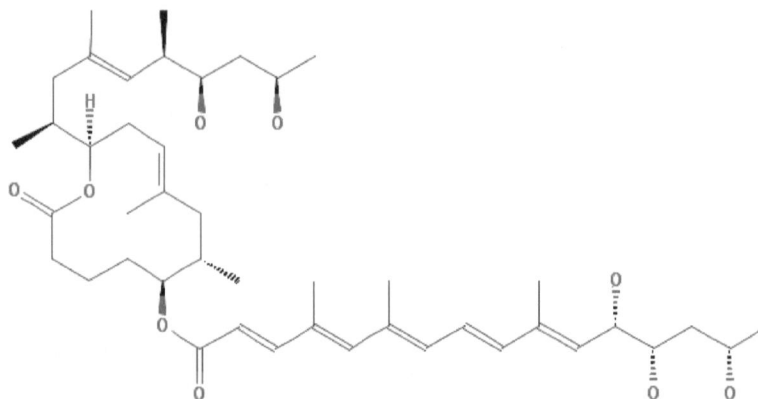

Figure 1: Chemical structure of mycolactone (PubChem Substance deposited record SID14298).

365 nm (UV-A) and a light intensity of 3 mW/cm^2, the half-life was just below 20 min (corresponding to 3 J/cm^2). Long-term exposure (6 h) eliminated all traces of ML, suggesting that the light completely disintegrated the molecule. The investigators reported loss of cytotoxic activity in parallel with the loss of material, confirming our own upublished data. In contrast, Xing et al found that exposure of ML in acetone to sunlight or light of 365 nm caused isomerization and cyclization of ML, accompanied by reduced cytotoxicity (Xing et al., 2012). The authors commented that their identified photomycolactone isomers could not be seen in disclosed spectroscopic data (MS, ^{1}H-NMR) from the study by Marion et al. This apparent discrepancy can perhaps be reconciled by assuming that Xing et al. in their experiments used light of low intensity, which caused isomerization but only limited disintegration.

ML appears to be metabolically stable and can be recovered from circulating blood cells and lymphoid organs of infected animal (Hong et al., 2008). Similar observations have been made also in BU patients, who have ML concentrations measurable by chromatography and mass spectroscopy (HPLC-MS/MS) in lesions, serum and ulcer exudate (Sarfo et al., 2010; Sarfo et al., 2011). The quantity of ML in serum of infected animals during infection is sufficient for detection of immunosuppressive activity (Hong et al., 2008; Phillips et al., 2009), and has been suggest to be responsible for the general immunosuppression seen in infected patients (Phillips et al., 2009). Interestingly, ML could be measured in ulcer exudates at the end of the antibiotic treatment period (Sarfo et al., 2010), suggesting a long half-life and persistence even after resolution of the infection.

3.2   Biological

Originally described as a cytotoxin, ML has several interesting effects also at nontoxic concentrations, the majority of them characterized in studies on immune cells. From these studies, it is clear that MU has developed mechanisms of immunosuppression, which appear to play an important role in the development of BU.

Experimental infection of animals has shown that phagocytic cells take up MU and migrate to draining lymph nodes (Coutanceau et al., 2005). MU multiplies inside cultured mouse macrophages when using low multiplicities of infection to prevent early ML-associated cytotoxicity (Torrado et al., 2007). Following the proliferation phase within macrophages, MU induces the lysis of the infected host cells and

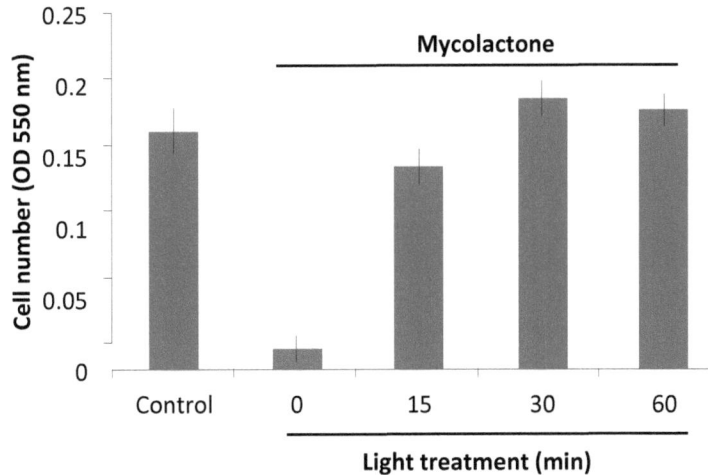

Figure 2: Mycolactone is sensitive to sunlight. Mycolactone in polypropylene vials was kept in the dark (0 min) or exposed to sunlight for 15-60 min, and thereafter tested for cytotoxicity on cultured Calu-6 cells at 300 ng/ml. Cell numbers were measured after 24 h at 37°C, 5% CO_2 by staining with neutral red and measuring optical density at 550 nm.

thus become extracellular. Released ML inhibits further phagocytosis by macrophages and alters the inflammatory response by inhibiting the production of inflammatory cytokines like TNF-α and up-regulating inflammatory cytokines like MIP-2 (Coutanceau *et al.*, 2005; Torrado *et al.*, 2007). Even if there is a constant influx of inflammatory cells to sites of active infection, these may be killed by ML. In spite of this, there is evidence of ongoing inflammatory and immunological reactions in infected tissue (Peduzzi *et al.*, 2007). However, bacterial production of ML may inhibit the initiation of primary immune responses via its ability to inhibit the recruitment of antigen presenting dendritic cells, and selectively modulate their cytokine/chemokine repertoire (Coutanceau *et al.*, 2007).

Defective cell-mediated immunity measured as production of cytokines following stimulation with mycobacterial antigens and other antigens, is demonstrable in patients with active BU (Gooding *et al.*, 2001; Gooding *et al.*, 2002; Yeboah-Manu *et al.*, 2006; Phillips *et al.*, 2009). In particular, production of IFN-γ is down-modulated, indicating a defective cell-mediated (Th1) immune response during active infection. In an experimental mouse model of infection, Fraga *et al.*, (Fraga *et al.*, 2011), demonstrated that spread of MU to draining lymph nodes gave rise to increased apoptosis and depletion of antigen specific, IFN-γproducing, CD4[+] T cells. The number of IFN-γ producing cells against non-mycobacterial antigens is also reduced in BU patients but recovers after surgical treatment (Yeboah-Manu *et al.*, 2006). In contrast, the majority of patients produce cytokines associated with a Th2-type humoral response. In support of this, the presence of antibodies to MU also in individuals who have no history of BU, indicates that infection can occur without disease development (Gooding *et al.*, 2001). In fact, only a subgroup of infected individuals are considered to show overt signs of infection (Schutte & Pluschke 2009).

4   Pathogenic Role of Mycolactone

ML has evolved in MU as a multi-functional cytotoxin increasing the chances of MU to survive in infected host species. At the cellular level, ML cytotoxicity probably has a role in release and spread of intracellular growing bacteria (Rondini et al., 2006). It can be envisaged that a high local concentration of ML destroys nearby tissue cells thus causing ulceration, and may also kill immune cells. At low, non-toxic concentrations of ML, its immunosuppressive effects on white blood cells may prevent an immunological response from effective initiation and propagation. ML also has demonstrable cytopathic effects on muscle tissue, which may lead to weakness and atrophy (Houngbedji et al., 2011). A similar effect on nerve cells may explain the lack of pain in BU (Goto et al., 2006; En et al., 2008).

Recent studies, described below, shed light on several parallel molecular mechanisms of ML action. These may be more or less cell type specific and concentration dependent, but appear to provide plausible molecular explanations for how ML exerts its pathogenic effects.

4.1   Cytotoxicity

ML is cytotoxic to epithelial (Bozzo et al., 2010; Gronberg et al., 2010), adipose cells (Dobos et al., 2001), fibroblasts (George et al., 1999) and monocytes (George et al., 2000). Fibroblasts and keratinocytes are killed by low (ng/ml) concentrations, while some cell lines are more resistant (Bozzo et al., 2010). At the cellular level, ML induces alterations in the cytoskeleton of cells followed by arrest in the G_0/G_1 phase of the cell cycle and eventually mediates cell death by apoptosis (George et al., 2000).

Keratinocyte cell death induced by ML is associated with production of reactive oxygen species (ROS) and can be inhibited by antioxidants (Gronberg et al., 2010). Inhibition of cell death by the iron chelating substance deferoxamine, suggests that ROS production involves Fe^{2+}-dependent production of hydroxyl radicals. Hydroxyl radicals would normally be toxic for bacteria and act as a defense mechanism against intracellular parasites. However, there may be concentrations at which the bacteria in the phagosome can utilize iron for their intracellular growth and still resist the hostile environment resulting from iron oxidation. MU has active catalase and superoxide dismutase (Roberts & Hirst 1996), which may aid in resistance to host cell derived ROS.

The utilization of iron for intracellular growth appears to be an important feature shared between the intracellular parasites MU and M. tuberculosis as suggested by the role of iron transport proteins in these diseases. Increased availability of iron usually results in increased growth of *M. tuberculosis* in vitro (Youdim 1969) and in vivo (Kochan 1973) and iron depletion by administration of an iron chelator like deferoxamine reduces their growth (Schaible et al., 2002).

The protein NRAMP1 (SLC11A1) is mediating transport of divalent cations across the phagosomal membrane and plays an important role in resistance against infection by intracellular parasites like mycobacteria (Goswami et al., 2001). The prevailing view is that NRAMP1 is responsible for Fe^{2+} efflux from the phagosome, thereby restricting bacterial growth (Stienstra et al., 2006; Boelaert et al., 2007; Cellier et al., 2007). Susceptibility to BU is associated with a D543N polymorphism in NRAMP1 with an odds ratio of 2.66 (Stienstra et al., 2006). A similar association for this polymorphism has been reported for tuberculosis with an odds ratio of 1.67. Additional polymorphic loci in this gene have been reported to increase the risk of pulmonary tuberculosis (Awomoyi et al., 2002; Li et al., 2006).

Taken together, the roles of iron, iron transport and production of ROS in BU pathology provide interesting topics for further investigations and may provide support for clinical testing of an iron chelator such as deferoxamine as an adjunct to antibiotic treatment.

4.2   Inhibition of Cell Functions

Several recent studies have unraveled specific interference by ML with intracellular signal transduction and regulatory mechanisms. These effects occur at non-toxic concentrations of ML and are not directly responsible for its cytotoxic effect but may, via a common pathway, converge into cell death at high ML concentrations.

Uptake of ML is both non-saturable and non-competitive, consistent with passive diffusion of this toxin through the cell membrane and compatible with a cytosolic target for ML (Snyder & Small 2003).

ML mediates inhibition of IL-6 production in primary human monocytes by reducing mRNA translation. This mechanism is distinct from rapamycin, another naturally occurring immunosuppressive lactone (Simmonds et al., 2009). It was subsequently shown in T cells that ML triggered lipid-raft association and activation of the Src-family kinase Lck (Boulkroun et al., 2010). Lck is associated with CD4 and CD8 in T cells and plays a role in T cell activation (Veillette et al., 1991). ML-mediated hyperactivation of Lck resulted in the depletion of intracellular calcium stores and downregulation of T cell receptors, leading to impaired T cell responsiveness (Boulkroun et al., 2010).

Injection of ML into mice downregulated the adhesion molecule CD62L (L-selectin) on CD4[+] T cells, impaired their homing to lymph nodes and caused local cellular depletion (Guenin-Mace et al., 2011). The data indicated that the loss of CD62L occured without cell surface shedding but mainly post-transcriptionally, implicating a micro RNA, let-7b, as a regulator.

Studies of epithelial cells showed that ML disrupted autoinhibitory activity of the Wiscott-Aldrich syndrome protein (WASP), leading to activation of actin in the cytoplasm followed by defective cell adhesion and directional migration (Guenin-Mace et al., 2013)..

An interesting possibility warranting further investigations is that the described effects on Lck and WASP are somehow related to increased ROS production triggered by ML. ROS, H_2O_2 in particular, are well-established signaling molecules and have been reported to be involved in regulation of Lck and WASP pathways (Hardwick & Sefton 1995; Taulet et al., 2012). Downregulation of CD62L expression is also reported to occur via ROS. However, this effect is usually mediated via proteolytic cleavage and shedding of CD62L (Wang et al., 2009), a phenomenon which did not take place in T cells treated with ML.

5   Mycolactone as a Therapeutic Target

MU pathology is governed by a unique set of genes and proteins that may serve as targets for new drugs to treat this disease (Butt et al., 2012). Given all observations pointing at the importance of ML in BU, it clearly represents a target in the development of improved therapies. There are several means described below by which this could be achieved.

5.1   Antibiotics and Antimicrobials

High ML production is associated with bacterial growth and reduced growth during the recommended antibiotic treatment leads to diminished ML (Sarfo et al., 2011; Sarfo et al., 2013). In the search for new effective oral combinations of antibiotics it may therefore be important to investigate their effect not only on the clearing of the infection, but also how they influence ML production. Alternatively, it may be possible to identify potent and selective inhibitors of the polyketide synthases that are responsible for ML synthesis in MU. If ML is as important as it seems in preventing an efficient elimination by the adaptive immune system, such an inhibitor may be sufficient for initiation of an effective cellular immune response.

5.2   Immunotherapy

There is as yet no specific vaccine against MU. BCG vaccination has been shown to offer some degree of protection against osteomyelitis (Portaels et al., 2002). BCG scar positive individuals with BU are also less inclined to develop metastatic ulcers than BCG scar negative BU patients (S. Britton, unpublished observation). Animal experiments have demonstrated delayed onset of ulcerative disease after vaccination with BCG or a ML negative strain of MU (Fraga et al., 2012). The prospect of being able to develop an effective vaccine is therefore promising (Huygen et al., 2009).

The development of an immune response after vaccination with ML is another possibility. However, attempts to create an immunogenic ML conjugate have apparently been unsuccessful (Schutte & Pluschke 2009). Alternatively it might be possible to use passive immunotherapy with monoclonal anti-ML antibodies, locally in the ulcer, or systemically.

5.3   Antioxidants

If generation of ROS is a central mechanism of ML´s effects, it may be possible to treat a diagnosed infection with high doses of antioxidants. The effect of deferoxamine could be tested in an experimental animal model of MU infection to test the hypothesis that iron oxidation is involved in the generation of ROS. If proven effective, it could provide a relatively safe, readily accessible and inexpensive drug for adjunct therapy together with antibiotics.

5.4   Phototherapy

The experimental data showing that ML was inactivated and destroyed by a relatively short exposure to sunlight, or filtered light of defined wavelength(s), suggest that local phototherapy may reduce the amount of ML present in an infected ulcer. Challenges that remain to be investigated are how ML is distributed in the ulcer tissue and how far the light penetrates through exudate, cells and extracellular matrix. In particular, the characteristically undermined ulcer edges that often occur in BU may prevent the light from reaching the entire ulcer area.

We have performed a pilot study with the aim to evaluate the effects of exposure to ultraviolet rays and visible light on experimental infection. BALB/c mice, divided into three groups, were inoculated intradermally in the footpad with MU^2, according to an established model (Fenner 1956; Sarfo et al., 2013). One group was exposed to ultraviolet UV-A light; one group to visible fluorescent light and a third group received no light treatment. Examination of the foot diameter and estimates of the extent of swelling and infection twice weekly did not reveal any significant differences in the progress of the disease found between the groups (Figure 2). This preliminary study suggests that exposure of MU lesions in mice to visible light and ultraviolet rays using this protocol had little or no effect on the progression of infection and inflammation. However, most of the lesions in this experiment did not consist of open ulcers. Therefore additional studies incorporating more controlled doses of light of different wavelengths and measurement of lesional levels of ML in open ulcers are required before any definite conclusions can be drawn.

The guinea-pig model of BU may be more useful than the mouse footpad model to study the effects of light exposure. In the former model, the bacteria are inoculated intradermally on the back of the animals, and developing ulcers can be exposed to direct light.

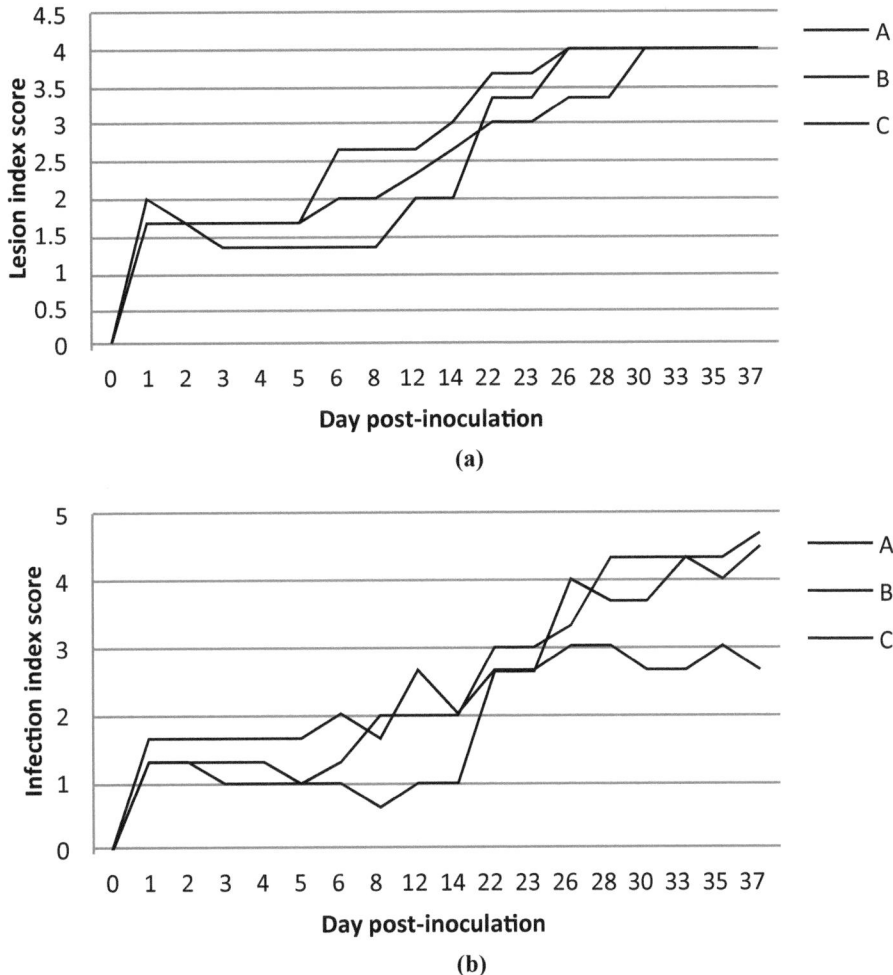

(a)

(b)

Figure 3: Light treatment of experimental *MU* lesions. Mice (N=3) were inoculated intradermally in their left hind footpad with (a) 7.5 μg mycolactone, or (b) 5 x 10^{10} CFU *MU.* From day 6, the inoculated feet were exposed to UV-A (A) from a portable lamp (Waldmann UV 109 A), or visible light (B) from a fluorescent light source, for 15 minutes a day, 5 days a week (C=control group). Average values of foot lesion swelling index scores are shown in (a), and infection index scores in (b).

Cope *et al.* (Cope *et al.*, 2002) showed that exposure to UV-B before inoculation with *MU* enhanced the infection in guinea pigs. Irradiation of mice with UV-R (with 65% UVB) before inoculation with other mycobacteria has previously been observed to impair the immune response against infection (Jeevan *et al.*, 1992; Jeevan *et al.*, 1995). Yet, light therapy is an established method against skin tuberculosis (Finsen & Forchhammer 1904) with a possible role played by vitamin D, an important modulator of the immune system, which synthesis is dependent on solar UV radiation,.

6   Conclusions

A relatively effective but cumbersome pharmacological combination protocol has since almost 10 years been in use in the treatment of BU, which is the third largest mycobacterial disease. The therapy is evolving towards new oral combinations of antibiotics, which hopefully will provide good cure and few side effects. We have highlighted the central role of ML in the disease and have described possible strategies for interference with ML or its effects that might provide starting points in the development of adjunct therapeutic protocols or new single drug therapies.

References

Adusumilli, S., Mve-Obiang, A., Sparer, T., Meyers, W., Hayman, J. & Small, P. L. (2005). *Mycobacterium ulcerans toxic macrolide, mycolactone modulates the host immune response and cellular location of M. ulcerans in vitro and in vivo. Cellular Microbiology 7(9): 1295-1304.*

Awomoyi, A. A., Marchant, A., Howson, J. M., McAdam, K. P., Blackwell, J. M. & Newport, M. J. (2002). *Interleukin-10, polymorphism in SLC11A1 (formerly NRAMP1), and susceptibility to tuberculosis. The Journal of infectious diseases 186(12): 1808-1814.*

Boelaert, J. R., Vandecasteele, S. J., Appelberg, R. & Gordeuk, V. R. (2007). *The effect of the host's iron status on tuberculosis. The Journal of infectious diseases 195(12): 1745-1753.*

Boulkroun, S., Guenin-Mace, L., Thoulouze, M. I., Monot, M., Merckx, A., Langsley, G., Bismuth, G., Di Bartolo, V. & Demangel, C. (2010). *Mycolactone suppresses T cell responsiveness by altering both early signaling and posttranslational events. Journal of Immunology 184(3): 1436-1444.*

Bozzo, C., Tiberio, R., Graziola, F., Pertusi, G., Valente, G., Colombo, E., Small, P. L. & Leigheb, G. (2010). *A Mycobacterium ulcerans toxin, mycolactone, induces apoptosis in primary human keratinocytes and in HaCaT cells. Microbes and Infection / Institut Pasteur 12(14-15): 1258-1263.*

Butt, A. M., Nasrullah, I., Tahir, S. & Tong, Y. (2012). *Comparative genomics analysis of Mycobacterium ulcerans for the identification of putative essential genes and therapeutic candidates. PloS one 7(8): e43080.*

Cellier, M. F., Courville, P. & Campion, C. (2007). *Nramp1 phagocyte intracellular metal withdrawal defense. Microbes and Infection / Institut Pasteur 9(14-15): 1662-1670.*

Chauty, A., Ardant, M. F., Marsollier, L., Pluschke, G., Landier, J., Adeye, A., Goundote, A., Cottin, J., Ladikpo, T., Ruf, T. & Ji, B. (2011). *Oral treatment for Mycobacterium ulcerans infection: results from a pilot study in Benin. Clinical Infectious Diseases : an official publication of the Infectious Diseases Society of America 52(1): 94-96.*

Clancey, J. K., Dodge, O. G., Lunn, H. F. & Oduori, M. L. (1961). *Mycobacterial skin ulcers in Uganda. Lancet 2(7209): 951-954.*

Connor, D. H. & Lunn, H. F. (1966). *A clinicopathologic study of 38 Ugandans with Mycobacterium ulcerans ulceration. Archives in Pathology 81: 183.*

Cope, R. B., Hartman, J. A., Morrow, C. K., Haschek, W. M. & Small, P. L. (2002). Ultraviolet radiation enhances both the nodular and ulcerative forms of Mycobacterium ulcerans infection in a Crl:IAF(HA)-hrBR hairless guinea pig model of Buruli ulcer disease. Photodermatology, photoimmunology & photomedicine 18(6): 271-279.

Coutanceau, E., Decalf, J., Martino, A., Babon, A., Winter, N., Cole, S. T., Albert, M. L. & Demangel, C. (2007). Selective suppression of dendritic cell functions by Mycobacterium ulcerans toxin mycolactone. Journal of Experimental Medicine 204(6): 1395-1403.

Coutanceau, E., Marsollier, L., Brosch, R., Perret, E., Goossens, P., Tanguy, M., Cole, S. T., Small, P. L. & Demangel, C. (2005). Modulation of the host immune response by a transient intracellular stage of Mycobacterium ulcerans: the contribution of endogenous mycolactone toxin. Cellular Microbiology 7(8): 1187-1196.

Dega, H., Bentoucha, A., Robert, J., Jarlier, V. & Grosset, J. (2002). Bactericidal activity of rifampin-amikacin against Mycobacterium ulcerans in mice. Antimicrobial agents and chemotherapy 46(10): 3193-3196.

Dega, H., Robert, J., Bonnafous, P., Jarlier, V. & Grosset, J. (2000). Activities of several antimicrobials against Mycobacterium ulcerans infection in mice. Antimicrobial agents and chemotherapy 44(9): 2367-2372.

Dobos, K. M., Small, P. L., Deslauriers, M., Quinn, F. D. & King, C. H. (2001). Mycobacterium ulcerans cytotoxicity in an adipose cell model. Infection and Immunity 69(11): 7182-7186.

En, J., Goto, M., Nakanaga, K., Higashi, M., Ishii, N., Saito, H., Yonezawa, S., Hamada, H. & Small, P. L. (2008). Mycolactone is responsible for the painlessness of Mycobacterium ulcerans infection (buruli ulcer) in a murine study. Infection and Immunity 76(5): 2002-2007.

Etuaful, S., Carbonnelle, B., Grosset, J., Lucas, S., Horsfield, C., Phillips, R., Evans, M., Ofori-Adjei, D., Klustse, E., Owusu-Boateng, J., Amedofu, G. K., Awuah, P., Ampadu, E., Amofah, G., Asiedu, K. & Wansbrough-Jones, M. (2005). Efficacy of the combination rifampin-streptomycin in preventing growth of Mycobacterium ulcerans in early lesions of Buruli ulcer in humans. Antimicrobial agents and chemotherapy 49(8): 3182-3186.

Fenner, F. (1956). The pathogenic behavior of Mycobacterium ulcerans and Mycobacterium balnei in the mouse and the developing chick embryo. American review of tuberculosis 73(5): 650-673.

Finsen, N. R. & Forchhammer, H. (1904). Resultate der Lichtbehandlung bei unseren ersten 800 Fällen von Lupus vulgaris. Mitteilungen aus Finsen's Medizinischer Lichtinstitut 5/6: 1–48.

Fraga, A. G., Cruz, A., Martins, T. G., Torrado, E., Saraiva, M., Pereira, D. R., Meyers, W. M., Portaels, F., Silva, M. T., Castro, A. G. & Pedrosa, J. (2011). Mycobacterium ulcerans triggers T-cell immunity followed by local and regional but not systemic immunosuppression. Infection and Immunity 79(1): 421-430.

Fraga, A. G., Martins, T. G., Torrado, E., Huygen, K., Portaels, F., Silva, M. T., Castro, A. G. & Pedrosa, J. (2012). Cellular immunity confers transient protection in experimental Buruli ulcer following BCG or mycolactone-negative Mycobacterium ulcerans vaccination. PloS one 7(3): e33406.

George, K. M., Barker, L. P., Welty, D. M. & Small, P. L. (1998). Partial purification and characterization of biological effects of a lipid toxin produced by Mycobacterium ulcerans. Infection and Immunity 66(2): 587-593.

George, K. M., Chatterjee, D., Gunawardana, G., Welty, D., Hayman, J., Lee, R. & Small, P. L. (1999). Mycolactone: a polyketide toxin from Mycobacterium ulcerans required for virulence. Science 283(5403): 854-857.

George, K. M., Pascopella, L., Welty, D. M. & Small, P. L. (2000). A Mycobacterium ulcerans toxin, mycolactone, causes apoptosis in guinea pig ulcers and tissue culture cells. Infection and Immunity 68(2): 877-883.

Gooding, T. M., Johnson, P. D., Campbell, D. E., Hayman, J. A., Hartland, E. L., Kemp, A. S. & Robins-Browne, R. M. (2001). Immune response to infection with Mycobacterium ulcerans. Infect and Immunity 69(3): 1704-1707.

Gooding, T. M., Johnson, P. D., Smith, M., Kemp, A. S. & Robins-Browne, R. M. (2002). Cytokine profiles of patients infected with Mycobacterium ulcerans and unaffected household contacts. Infect and Immunity 70(10): 5562-5567.

Goswami, T., Bhattacharjee, A., Babal, P., Searle, S., Moore, E., Li, M. & Blackwell, J. M. (2001). Natural-resistance-associated macrophage protein 1 is an H+/bivalent cation antiporter. The Biochemical journal 354(Pt 3): 511-519.

Goto, M., Nakanaga, K., Aung, T., Hamada, T., Yamada, N., Nomoto, M., Kitajima, S., Ishii, N., Yonezawa, S. & Saito, H. (2006). Nerve damage in Mycobacterium ulcerans-infected mice: probable cause of painlessness in buruli ulcer. The American journal of pathology 168(3): 805-811.

Gronberg, A., Zettergren, L., Bergh, K., Stahle, M., Heilborn, J., Angeby, K., Small, P. L., Akuffo, H. & Britton, S. (2010). Antioxidants protect keratinocytes against M. ulcerans mycolactone cytotoxicity. PloS one 5(11): e13839.

Guenin-Mace, L., Carrette, F., Asperti-Boursin, F., Le Bon, A., Caleechurn, L., Di Bartolo, V., Fontanet, A., Bismuth, G. & Demangel, C. (2011). Mycolactone impairs T cell homing by suppressing microRNA control of L-selectin expression. Proceedings of the National Academy of Sciences of the United States of America 108(31): 12833-12838.

Guenin-Mace, L., Veyron-Churlet, R., Thoulouze, M. I., Romet-Lemonne, G., Hong, H., Leadlay, P. F., Danckaert, A., Ruf, M. T., Mostowy, S., Zurzolo, C., Bousso, P., Chretien, F., Carlier, M. F. & Demangel, C. (2013). Mycolactone activation of Wiskott-Aldrich syndrome proteins underpins Buruli ulcer formation. The Journal of clinical investigation 123(4): 1501-1512.

Hardwick, J. S. & Sefton, B. M. (1995). Activation of the Lck tyrosine protein kinase by hydrogen peroxide requires the phosphorylation of Tyr-394. Proceedings of the National Academy of Sciences of the United States of America 92(10): 4527-4531.

Hong, H., Coutanceau, E., Leclerc, M., Caleechurn, L., Leadlay, P. F. & Demangel, C. (2008). Mycolactone diffuses from Mycobacterium ulcerans-infected tissues and targets mononuclear cells in peripheral blood and lymphoid organs. PLoS neglected tropical diseases 2(10): e325.

Hong, H., Demangel, C., Pidot, S. J., Leadlay, P. F. & Stinear, T. (2008). Mycolactones: immunosuppressive and cytotoxic polyketides produced by aquatic mycobacteria. Natural product reports 25(3): 447-454.

Houngbedji, G. M., Bouchard, P. & Frenette, J. (2011). Mycobacterium ulcerans infections cause progressive muscle atrophy and dysfunction, and mycolactone impairs satellite cell proliferation. American journal of physiology. Regulatory, integrative and comparative physiology 300(3): R724-732.

Huygen, K., Adjei, O., Affolabi, D., Bretzel, G., Demangel, C., Fleischer, B., Johnson, R. C., Pedrosa, J., Phanzu, D. M., Phillips, R. O., Pluschke, G., Siegmund, V., Singh, M., van der Werf, T. S., Wansbrough-Jones, M. & Portaels, F. (2009). Buruli ulcer disease: prospects for a vaccine. Medical microbiology and immunology 198(2): 69-77.

Jeevan, A., Bucana, C. D., Dong, Z., Dizon, V. V., Thomas, S. L., Lloyd, T. E. & Kripke, M. L. (1995). Ultraviolet radiation reduces phagocytosis and intracellular killing of mycobacteria and inhibits nitric oxide production by macrophages in mice. Journal of Leukocyte Biology 57(6): 883-890.

Jeevan, A., Evans, R., Brown, E. L. & Kripke, M. L. (1992). Effect of local ultraviolet irradiation on infections of mice with Candida albicans, Mycobacterium bovis BCG, and Schistosoma mansoni. The Journal of Investigative Dermatology 99(1): 59-64.

Kibadi, K., Boelaert, M., Fraga, A. G., Kayinua, M., Longatto-Filho, A., Minuku, J. B., Mputu-Yamba, J. B., Muyembe-Tamfum, J. J., Pedrosa, J., Roux, J. J., Meyers, W. M. & Portaels, F. (2010). Response to treatment in a prospective cohort of patients with large ulcerated lesions suspected to be Buruli Ulcer (Mycobacterium ulcerans disease). PLoS neglected tropical diseases 4(7): e736.

Kochan, I. (1973). The role of iron in bacterial infections, with special consideration of host-tubercle bacillus interaction. Current topics in microbiology and immunology 60: 1-30.

Li, H. T., Zhang, T. T., Zhou, Y. Q., Huang, Q. H. & Huang, J. (2006). SLC11A1 (formerly NRAMP1) gene polymorphisms and tuberculosis susceptibility: a meta-analysis. The International Journal of Tuberculosis and Lung Disease 10(1): 3-12.

Lipman, M. & Breen, R. (2006). Immune reconstitution inflammatory syndrome in HIV. Current opinion in infectious diseases 19(1): 20-25.

MacCallum, P., Tolhurst, J. C., Buckle, G. & Sissons, H. A. (1948). A new mycobacterial infection in man. The Journal of pathology and bacteriology 60(1): 93-122.

Marion, E., Prado, S., Cano, C., Babonneau, J., Ghamrawi, S. & Marsollier, L. (2012). Photodegradation of the Mycobacterium ulcerans toxin, mycolactones: considerations for handling and storage. PloS one 7(4): e33600.

Marsollier, L., Robert, R., Aubry, J., Saint Andre, J. P., Kouakou, H., Legras, P., Manceau, A. L., Mahaza, C. & Carbonnelle, B. (2002). Aquatic insects as a vector for Mycobacterium ulcerans. Applied and environmental microbiology 68(9): 4623-4628.

Mve-Obiang, A., Lee, R. E., Portaels, F. & Small, P. L. (2003). Heterogeneity of mycolactones produced by clinical isolates of Mycobacterium ulcerans: implications for virulence. Infection and Immunology 71(2): 774-783.

Nienhuis, W. A., Stienstra, Y., Thompson, W. A., Awuah, P. C., Abass, K. M., Tuah, W., Awua-Boateng, N. Y., Ampadu, E. O., Siegmund, V., Schouten, J. P., Adjei, O., Bretzel, G. & van der Werf, T. S. (2010). Antimicrobial treatment for early, limited Mycobacterium ulcerans infection: a randomised controlled trial. Lancet 375(9715): 664-672.

O'Brien, D. P., Robson, M. E., Callan, P. P. & McDonald, A. H. (2009). "Paradoxical" immune-mediated reactions to Mycobacterium ulcerans during antibiotic treatment: a result of treatment success, not failure. The Medical journal of Australia 191(10): 564-566.

Oliveira, M. S., Fraga, A. G., Torrado, E., Castro, A. G., Pereira, J. P., Filho, A. L., Milanezi, F., Schmitt, F. C., Meyers, W. M., Portaels, F., Silva, M. T. & Pedrosa, J. (2005). Infection with Mycobacterium ulcerans induces persistent inflammatory responses in mice. Infection and Immunity 73(10): 6299-6310.

Peduzzi, E., Groeper, C., Schutte, D., Zajac, P., Rondini, S., Mensah-Quainoo, E., Spagnoli, G. C., Pluschke, G. & Daubenberger, C. A. (2007). Local activation of the innate immune system in Buruli ulcer lesions. Journal of Investigative Dermatology 127(3): 638-645.

Phillips, R., Sarfo, F. S., Guenin-Mace, L., Decalf, J., Wansbrough-Jones, M., Albert, M. L. & Demangel, C. (2009). Immunosuppressive signature of cutaneous Mycobacterium ulcerans infection in the peripheral blood of patients with buruli ulcer disease. The Journal of infectious diseases 200(11): 1675-1684.

Portaels, F., Aguiar, J., Debacker, M., Steunou, C., Zinsou, C., Guedenon, A. & Meyers, W. M. (2002). Prophylactic effect of mycobacterium bovis BCG vaccination against osteomyelitis in children with Mycobacterium ulcerans disease (Buruli Ulcer). Clinical and Diagnostic Laboratory Immunology 9(6): 1389-1391.

Roberts, B. & Hirst, R. (1996). Identification and characterisation of a superoxide dismutase and catalase from Mycobacterium ulcerans. Journal of medical microbiology 45(5): 383-387.

Rondini, S., Horsfield, C., Mensah-Quainoo, E., Junghanss, T., Lucas, S. & Pluschke, G. (2006). Contiguous spread of Mycobacterium ulcerans in Buruli ulcer lesions analysed by histopathology and real-time PCR quantification of mycobacterial DNA. The Journal of pathology 208(1): 119-128.

Sarfo, F. S., Converse, P. J., Almeida, D. V., Zhang, J., Robinson, C., Wansbrough-Jones, M. & Grosset, J. H. (2013). Microbiological, histological, immunological, and toxin response to antibiotic treatment in the mouse model of Mycobacterium ulcerans disease. PLoS neglected tropical diseases 7(3): e2101.

Sarfo, F. S., Le Chevalier, F., Aka, N., Phillips, R. O., Amoako, Y., Boneca, I. G., Lenormand, P., Dosso, M., Wansbrough-Jones, M., Veyron-Churlet, R., Guenin-Mace, L. & Demangel, C. (2011). Mycolactone diffuses into the peripheral blood of Buruli ulcer patients--implications for diagnosis and disease monitoring. PLoS neglected tropical diseases 5(7): e1237.

Sarfo, F. S., Phillips, R., Asiedu, K., Ampadu, E., Bobi, N., Adentwe, E., Lartey, A., Tetteh, I. & Wansbrough-Jones, M. (2010). Clinical efficacy of combination of rifampin and streptomycin for treatment of Mycobacterium ulcerans disease. Antimicrobial agents and chemotherapy 54(9): 3678-3685.

Sarfo, F. S., Phillips, R. O., Rangers, B., Mahrous, E. A., Lee, R. E., Tarelli, E., Asiedu, K. B., Small, P. L. & Wansbrough-Jones, M. H. (2010). Detection of Mycolactone A/B in Mycobacterium ulcerans-Infected Human Tissue. PLoS neglected tropical diseases 4(1): e577.

Schaible, U. E., Collins, H. L., Priem, F. & Kaufmann, S. H. (2002). Correction of the iron overload defect in beta-2-microglobulin knockout mice by lactoferrin abolishes their increased susceptibility to tuberculosis. The Journal of Experimental Medicine 196(11): 1507-1513.

Schutte, D. & Pluschke, G. (2009). *Immunosuppression and treatment-associated inflammatory response in patients with Mycobacterium ulcerans infection (Buruli ulcer). Expert opinion on biological therapy 9(2): 187-200.*

Simmonds, R. E., Lali, F. V., Smallie, T., Small, P. L. C. & Foxwell, B. M. (2009). *Mycolactone Inhibits Monocyte Cytokine Production by a Posttranscriptional Mechanism. Journa of Immunology 182(4): 2194-2202.*

Snyder, D. S. & Small, P. L. (2003). *Uptake and cellular actions of mycolactone, a virulence determinant for Mycobacterium ulcerans. Microbial pathogenesis 34(2): 91-101.*

Stienstra, Y., van der Werf, T. S., Oosterom, E., Nolte, I. M., van der Graaf, W. T., Etuaful, S., Raghunathan, P. L., Whitney, E. A., Ampadu, E. O., Asamoa, K., Klutse, E. Y., te Meerman, G. J., Tappero, J. W., Ashford, D. A. & van der Steege, G. (2006). *Susceptibility to Buruli ulcer is associated with the SLC11A1 (NRAMP1) D543N polymorphism. Genes and immunity 7(3): 185-189.*

Stienstra, Y., van Roest, M. H., van Wezel, M. J., Wiersma, I. C., Hospers, I. C., Dijkstra, P. U., Johnson, R. C., Ampadu, E. O., Gbovi, J., Zinsou, C., Etuaful, S., Klutse, E. Y., van der Graaf, W. T. & van der Werf, T. S. (2005). *Factors associated with functional limitations and subsequent employment or schooling in Buruli ulcer patients. Tropical Medicine & International Health 10(12): 1251-1257.*

Stinear, T. P., Mve-Obiang, A., Small, P. L., Frigui, W., Pryor, M. J., Brosch, R., Jenkin, G. A., Johnson, P. D., Davies, J. K., Lee, R. E., Adusumilli, S., Garnier, T., Haydock, S. F., Leadlay, P. F. & Cole, S. T. (2004). *Giant plasmid-encoded polyketide synthases produce the macrolide toxin of Mycobacterium ulcerans. Proc Natl Acad Sci U S A 101(5): 1345-1349.*

Taulet, N., Delorme-Walker, V. D. & DerMardirossian, C. (2012). *Reactive oxygen species regulate protrusion efficiency by controlling actin dynamics. PloS one 7(8): e41342.*

Torrado, E., Adusumilli, S., Fraga, A. G., Small, P. L., Castro, A. G. & Pedrosa, J. (2007). *Mycolactone-mediated inhibition of tumor necrosis factor production by macrophages infected with Mycobacterium ulcerans has implications for the control of infection. Infection and Immunity 75(8): 3979-3988.*

Torrado, E., Fraga, A. G., Castro, A. G., Stragier, P., Meyers, W. M., Portaels, F., Silva, M. T. & Pedrosa, J. (2007). *Evidence for an intramacrophage growth phase of Mycobacterium ulcerans. Infection and Immunity 75(2): 977-987.*

Veillette, A., Abraham, N., Caron, L. & Davidson, D. (1991). *The lymphocyte-specific tyrosine protein kinase p56lck. Seminars in immunology 3(3): 143-152.*

Wade, H. W. (1955). *A tuberculoid-like reaction in lepromatous leprosy; a reactional reversal phenomenon. International journal of Leprosy 23(4 Part 1): 443-446.*

Wang, Y., Herrera, A. H., Li, Y., Belani, K. K. & Walcheck, B. (2009). *Regulation of mature ADAM17 by redox agents for L-selectin shedding. Journal of Immunology 182(4): 2449-2457.*

Xing, Y., Hande, S. M. & Kishi, Y. (2012). *Photochemistry of mycolactone A/B, the causative toxin of Buruli ulcer. Journal of the American Chemical Society 134(46): 19234-19239.*

Yeboah-Manu, D., Peduzzi, E., Mensah-Quainoo, E., Asante-Poku, A., Ofori-Adjei, D., Pluschke, G. & Daubenberger, C. A. (2006). *Systemic suppression of interferon-gamma responses in Buruli ulcer patients resolves after surgical excision of the lesions caused by the extracellular pathogen Mycobacterium ulcerans. Journal of Leukocyte Biology 79(6): 1150-1156.*

Youdim, S. (1969). *In vitro effect of iron salts and chelating agents on serum tuberculostasis. The American review of respiratory disease 99(6): 925-931.*

www.ingramcontent.com/pod-product-compliance
Lightning Source LLC
Chambersburg PA
CBHW041445210326
41599CB00004B/134